Health Guide

The ultimate reference on how to live healthier, longer and happier

Version 1 (May 2024)

ISBN-13: 978-84-09-61163-8
Cover designed by Mariana Carsi

Content

Prologue

Health is one of the most precious things we have, if not the most.
Until we have health problems, we might not give it the deserved consideration and we may take it for granted.
What if, instead, you start by paying the right attention to it now?
Our healthy habits have a greater impact if we start working on them from the early beginning, and this is the central idea of the book on health prevention. Not only is a longer life expectancy desired, but so is an improved quality of life, which is the most fundamental difference between lifespan and healthspan.

Due to the breadth and depth of the topic, we often find ourselves unsure of how to act in order to carry out our everyday responsibilities appropriately. Many sources disseminate information, but its reliability is frequently called into question because it is based on personal opinion rather than solid evidence. This information might be inaccurate, imply theories without supporting facts, and even dangerous in some cases. The scientific and medical community suggest health guidelines, but they are scattered across the web and difficult for the average person to locate.

The goal of this book is to compile all this knowledge in a logical structure so you have a comprehensive and practical reference to the most important aspects of your health. Put simply, this book will teach you the little things you may do on a daily basis to improve the state of your mind and body.
The content is based on the principles aligned by the highest experts in the field, from national and international organizations like the World Health Organization and the Centers for Disease Control and Prevention, to medical societies and foundations like the Hearth Association. If these

sources do not provide enough concrete information, other reputable sources like Harvard are also consulted.
The book's methodology also selects the health topics in a ranked order of importance according to how common they are, how they affect our lives, and how dangerous they could be.
Moreover, most of the principles focus on prevention, so not in diagnosis or treatment, because it's expected that these steps are already covered widely by the healthcare system. The only exceptions have been taken on first aid, to understand better what you can do while waiting for the healthcare providers, and over-the-counter remedies, namely those that do not require a prescription, in order to avoid their improper use.

After reading this book, nobody expects you to suddenly transform into a lifestyle model example and adhere rigidly to all of these rules, however you will have the power of knowledge and be able to make informed decisions about the changes you want to make in your life.
You can gradually incorporate these changes, finding the right balance on setting a realistic lifestyle, that you can implement with constancy in the long term.
You will not find a miracle recipe or magic formula here, but "just" the reliable alignments that medical societies identify.

Who am I?
I am a biomedical engineer, graduated in one of the best universities in Italy. After several years of work experience in the healthcare sector and earning an MBA from a global top-10 business school, I am currently an executive in one of the largest pharma companies in the world.
As a professional who has overseen patient support programs, I have seen firsthand how a patient's lifestyle, level of engagement, and amount of misinformation affect clinical outcomes.
After reading books on the different aspects of healthy habits (i.e. nutrition, sports, meditation, respiration), I have noticed that there was not yet a complete reference covering all of them in the same book and including clear actions the reader can take.

That's why I have decided to write this book, with the hope of contributing with a small drop to this ocean of mankind's health.

Enjoy your read, and be healthy, be happy!

Disclaimer

No content in this book should ever be used as a substitute for direct medical advice from your doctor or other qualified clinician. This is not clinical advice, and I do not assume the responsibility for potential harm due to these health guidelines.

Life expectancy

"I'm not afraid of death; I just don't want to be there when it happens".
Woody Allen (filmmaker and actor)

When and where[1]

Life expectancy is the best way to measure population health, and it has been going up quickly since the Age of Enlightenment in the 1700s. A big reason for it is that child mortality has decreased a lot during that time, but people of all ages can expect to live longer. This huge increase is due to many health improvements, such as better nutrition, clean water, sanitation, neonatal care, antibiotics, vaccines, technologies, and public health measures. It is also due to higher living standards, economic growth, and less poverty.

---

[1] UN World Population Prospects - https://ourworldindata.org/life-expectancy (Accessed in May 2024)

Year	World Life expectancy at birth (years)
1770	28.5
1800	28.5
1820	29.0
1850	29.3
1870	29.7
1900	32.0
1913	34.1
1950	46.5
1970	56.1
1990	64.0
2000	66.5
2010	70.1
2020	72.0

Life expectancy started to rise in the first developed countries in the early 1800s but stayed low in the rest of the world. This caused a huge difference in how health was spread around the world: good health in the wealthy nations and constant bad health in the poor nations, however, this **world inequality** has gone down over the last few decades. No country in the world has a lower life expectancy than the countries with the highest life expectancy in 1800.

The average life expectancy around the world has more than doubled since 1900 and is now over 70 years, and people in many of the world's richest countries can expect to live more than 80 years. In 2019, people in Spain, Switzerland, Italy, and Australia could expect to live more than 83 years. Japan achieved the highest, with almost 85 years. In the U.S., up to half of today's 5-year-olds are projected to live until 100 years old.

On the other side, people in the countries with the worst health can expect to live between 50 and 60 years. In 2019, people in the Central African Republic are expected to live the least, with only 53 years.[2]

[2] Stanford - https://news.stanford.edu/report/2022/08/16/wonderful-opportunity-rethinking-lifes-stages (Published in August 2022)

Another difference in life span is related to **gender**, since women generally live longer than men. This difference in life expectancy added up to 5 years in 2021: the average life expectancy for men was 68.4 years and the average life expectancy for women was 73.8 years. This difference starts at birth: newborn boys are more likely to die than girls because they are more likely to get diseases and genetic problems. It keeps happening when people are young, when boys are more likely to die than girls, usually because of accidents and violence. It stays the same as people get older, when men are more likely than women to die from long-term illnesses, partly because men are more likely to smoke, drink, and use drugs.[3]

Top causes of death[4-5]

Keeping track of how many people die each year helps to figure out how well our health care services are and where to put resources.
55% of the 55.4 million deaths that happened around the world in 2019 were caused by these top 10 diseases.

[3] Our World in Data - https://ourworldindata.org/why-do-women-live-longer-than-men (Published in November 2023)
[4] World Health Organization - https://www.who.int/news-room/fact-sheets/detail/the-top-10-causes-of-death (Published in December 2020)
[5] World Health Organization - https://www.who.int/news/item/09-12-2020-who-reveals-leading-causes-of-death-and-disability-worldwide-2000-2019 (Published in December 2020)

Leading causes of death globally	Number of deaths (millions)
Ischemic heart disease	8.9
Stroke	6.2
Chronic obstructive pulmonary disease	3.2
Lower respiratory infections	2.6
Neonatal conditions	2.0
Trachea, bronchus, lung cancers	1.8
Alzheimer disease and other dementias	1.6
Diarrheal diseases	1.5
Diabetes mellitus	1.5
Kidney diseases	1.3

Heart disease still kills more people than anything else: for the past 20 years, heart illness has been the main cause of death around the world, but currently it's killing more people than ever before. The number of deaths from heart disease increased by more than 2 million since 2000, to nearly 9 million in 2019.

Meanwhile diabetes and dementia are also now in the top 10. Between 2000 and 2019, the number of deaths from diabetes rose by 70% around the world.

Now let's make a comparison between the two opposite realities of the world, **low- versus high-income countries**, where we can see quite big differences on the causes of death.

Leading causes of death in low-income countries	**Number of deaths (hundred thousand)**
Neonatal conditions	5.2
Lower respiratory infections	4.1
Ischemic heart disease	3.9
Stroke	3.3
Diarrheal diseases	2.6
Malaria	2
Road injuries	2
Tuberculosis	1.8
HIV/AIDS	1.7
Cirrhosis of the liver	1

Leading causes of death in high-income countries	**Number of deaths (millions)**
Ischemic heart disease	1.7
Alzheimer disease and other dementias	0.8
Stroke	0.8
Trachea, bronchus, lung cancers	0.6
Chronic obstructive pulmonary disease	0.5
Lower respiratory infections	0.4
Colon and rectum cancers	0.3
Kidney diseases	0.3
Hypertensive heart disease	0.3
Diabetes mellitus	0.2

All but two of the top 10 diseases in high-income countries are killing more and more people, while **ischemic heart disease and stroke** are the only 2 that have seen a drop in deaths between 2000 and 2019, by 16% and 21% respectively. The only income group where the number of deaths from these two diseases has been going down is high-income.

There have been fewer deaths from **contagious diseases** around the world, but they are still a big problem in low- and middle-income countries. For example, HIV/AIDS dropped from the 8th most common cause of death in 2000 to the 19th in 2019. This shows how well efforts have been made over the last 20 years to prevent people from getting the virus, test for it, and treat it. The number of deaths has dropped by more than half, from over 1 million in 2000 to almost half a million in 2019, but it is still the 4th most common cause of death in Africa.

In the next chapters we will analyze most of these potential life threats, understanding the best ways to minimize the respective risks.

Take care of your heart[6]

The table from the last chapter shows that heart problems are the 1st and 2nd major causes of death around the world. This means that we should really think about how to take the best possible care of this organ.

The **heart** is about the size of your fist and works like a muscle pump. The heart is one of your most important muscles because it sends blood to all parts of your body. All of your cells need oxygen all the time.
Your heart is like a coordinated machine: your body's "used" blood is pumped by the right side of your heart to your lungs, where it gets oxygenated again, and then the left side of your heart sends this blood rich of oxygen back into your body. Your heart brings blood to almost every cell in your body. There are blood arteries that run through your body that are about 60,000 miles (96,000 km) long. In other words, this system of blood tubes could go around the Earth TWICE at the equator.
Your heart beats about 100,000 times every day, which means that the average person's heart beats more than 2.6 billion times before he/she dies. Your heart pumps about 5.7 liters (1.5 gallons) of blood every minute, and that's fast enough to fill an Olympic-sized pool in less than a year. About 8% of your body weight is blood. The lub-dub, lub-dub, lub-dub sound that comes from your heart is caused by valve leaflets

[6] American Heart Association - https://www.heart.org/en/health-topics/consumer-healthcare/what-is-cardiovascular-disease (Reviewed in January 2024)

opening and closing. Your heart has its own electrical supply, so it will keep beating even if it is not connected to your body.
To make room for your heart, your left lung is slightly smaller than your right lung.
Why does the heart stand for love? Most likely because of the pounding in your chest when Cupid's arrow hits you. But really, your brain feels love. That wouldn't make a good Valentine's Day sign, though.[7]

Cardiovascular diseases (CVDs), which are also known as heart and circulatory diseases, are a broad term for health problems that affect the heart or blood flow.
Heart attacks and strokes are generally acute events and are mostly caused by something blocking the flow of blood to the heart or brain. A buildup of fat on the inside walls or a blood clot in the blood vessels that bring blood to the heart or brain are the most common causes of this.

CVDs include the following:

- A **heart attack** happens when blood flow gets blocked to a part of the heart. If this block fully stops blood flow, the heart muscle that that artery serves will start to die. As a curiosity, the researchers found that the number of heart attacks went up noticeably at the start of the work week, and the number of heart attacks went up the most on Mondays by 13%. We still don't know the exact cause of this "Blue Monday" effect. It's heart attack season also during the holidays, since December 25 is the day of the year when the most heart-related deaths happen, and the 2nd and 3rd deadliest days are December 26 and January 1.
- **Ischemic strokes** occur when a blood vessel that brings blood to the brain gets blocked. When the blood flow gets cut off to a part of the brain, some brain cells will start to die because they can't get oxygen, and these cells are never renewed. The good

[7] Cleveland Clinic - https://health.clevelandclinic.org/fun-facts-about-your-heart (Published in August 2023)

news is that this kind of damage to brain cells doesn't always happen, and sometimes the damage is temporary.

- People often think that **heart failure** means the heart stops moving, but it actually means that the heart isn't pumping blood as well as it should. The heart keeps beating, but the body isn't getting the blood and oxygen it needs.
- If the heart beats too slowly, too quickly, or irregularly, that's **arrhythmia**. If the heart rate is less than 60 beats per minute, this is called bradycardia, and if it's higher than 100 it is tachycardia.
- **Atherosclerosis** is a condition that happens when plaque builds up in the walls of the arteries. It's harder for blood to flow through the arteries when this stuff builds up.

Heart cancer is very rare because heart cells stop growing when they reach adulthood. This makes them less likely to get mutations that can cause cancer.

At least 3 quarters of all CVD deaths happen in countries with **low or middle income**. People who live in low- and middle-income countries don't always have access to primary health care services that can find and treat people with CVD risk factors early on.

Bad fat [8]

Every cell in your body has **cholesterol** in it.
It's very important for your brain, muscles, skin, and in general the whole body. In addition to being a part of the membrane that covers all of your cells, cholesterol is also used to make vitamin D and steroid hormones that keep your bones, teeth, and muscles healthy. Finally, cholesterol is used to make bile, which breaks down fats you eat.

[8] Heart UK - https://www.heartuk.org.uk/cholesterol/what-is-cholesterol (Accessed in May 2024)

Even though our bodies need some cholesterol to work, having too much can block your arteries and cause health problems like heart disease in the future.

There isn't only cholesterol, but there are different kinds of **fats** that do different things to the body.
There are fats with **negative effects** on our bodies, such as:

- **LDL (Low-Density Lipoprotein) cholesterol** is often called "bad cholesterol". Too much LDL cholesterol can block your arteries and cause health problems like heart disease, heart attacks, and strokes in the future. There should be some LDL cholesterol in your blood, but while some cholesterol is good, too much of it can be harmful.
- **Triglycerides** are another kind of fat in the blood. Triglycerides are fats that get into your bloodstream after you eat them, and your liver also makes some of them. Along with cholesterol, triglycerides are packed into lipoproteins. When they get to your body's cells, they are either used as energy or saved for later.
  Getting your triglycerides checked at the same time as your cholesterol is a good idea. High triglycerides can be caused by a number of things, and it's important to figure out which one it is. When triglycerides are high, you may be more likely to get heart disease. If they're really high, they can also cause other major problems, like pancreatitis.[9]

From the other side, there are also fats with **positive effects**:

- **HDL (High-Density Lipoprotein) cholesterol**, or "good cholesterol", on the other hand, moves cholesterol from your cells to your liver to be broken down. It helps to prevent diseases.

---

[9] Harvard, School of Public Health - https://www.hsph.harvard.edu/nutritionsource/what-should-you-eat/fats-and-cholesterol/types-of-fat/omega-3-fats (Accessed in May 2024)

- More than half of the fats our bodies need can be made from other fats or carbs. **Omega 3** polyunsaturated fatty acids don't. They help make cell membranes all over the body and change how the cell receptors in these membranes work. They are also the building blocks for hormones that control inflammation, blood clotting, and the tightening and loosening of artery walls. They can also attach to receptors in cells that control how genes work. Therefore omega-3 fats may help keep you from getting heart disease and stroke, control lupus, eczema, and rheumatoid arthritis, and even protect against cancer and other diseases.

Which **values goal** of these fats is right for you depends on factors such as your age, health problems, and risk of cardiovascular disease.
The values below are guidelines for healthy adults, therefore, if you have a disease, take medication, or have recently had a child, your levels may be lower or higher.
Whether you have eaten something before the test does not have a significant effect on these values.

Type of cholesterol	mg/dL
Total cholesterol (TC)	below 193
Non-HDL cholesterol	below 155
LDL cholesterol	below 116
HDL cholesterol	above 39 for a man above 46 for a woman
TC:HDL ratio	Below 5
Triglyceride	below 150

The HDL cholesterol values in the table are considered the best precaution, but experts believe that there is no additional benefit to exceeding these values.

You may see the TC:HDL ratio, which is the ratio of HDL to total cholesterol, and this value should be as low as possible.[10]

As part of a healthy, balanced diet, most people do not need to lower the cholesterol levels of their foods, so you can continue to enjoy eggs and shellfish, but it is much more important to reduce your intake of foods that contain **saturated** fat. This is because saturated fat affects the way your liver processes cholesterol, therefore, consuming saturated fats can raise your cholesterol levels.

Cholesterol is only found in foods of animal origin - foods of plant origin do not contain cholesterol.

Foods that contain cholesterol and high levels of saturated fats.

- Full-fat dairy products such as milk, cheese, yogurt and cream.
- Animal fats such as butter, ghee, margarine and spreads made from animal fats, lard, tallow and drippings.
- Fatty meats and processed meat products such as sausages.

Try replacing saturated fats with heart-healthy **unsaturated fats** instead.

Foods that contain cholesterol but are low in saturated fat.

- Lean meat, especially offal such as liver, kidney, sweetbreads, hearts and tripe.
- Shrimp, crab, lobster, squid, octopus and cuttlefish.
- Eggs (cholesterol is in the yolk).[11]

Other foods also lower cholesterol in different ways.

Some provide soluble fiber, which binds cholesterol and its precursors in the digestive system and carries them out of the body before they enter the bloodstream. Some products provide polyunsaturated fats that directly lower LDL levels. Others contain plant sterols and stanols that block the absorption of cholesterol in the body.

---

[10] Heart UK - https://www.heartuk.org.uk/cholesterol/understanding-your-cholesterol-test-results- (Accessed in May 2024)

[11] Heart UK - https://www.heartuk.org.uk/low-cholesterol-foods/foods-that-contain-cholesterol (Accessed in May 2024)

- Oats: An easy first step to lowering cholesterol is to eat a bowl of oatmeal or an oatmeal-based cold cereal like Cheerios for breakfast. Current dietary guidelines recommend consuming 20-35 grams of fiber each day, with at least 5-10 grams coming from soluble fiber (the average American gets about half that).
- Barley and other whole grain products: Like oats and oat bran, barley and other whole grains provide mostly soluble fiber, which may help reduce the risk of heart disease.
- Beans: Beans are especially rich in soluble fiber, and in addition, it takes the body longer to digest them, which makes you feel fuller longer after a meal. This is one of the reasons why beans are a useful food for people who want to lose weight.
- Eggplant and okra: These two low-calorie vegetables are good sources of soluble fiber.
- Nuts: Numerous studies have shown that eating almonds, walnuts, peanuts, and other nuts is good for your heart. Eating 2 ounces (55 grams) of nuts per day can reduce LDL levels by about 5%. Nuts contain additional nutrients that protect your heart in another way.
- Vegetable oils: Using liquid vegetable oils such as canola, sunflower, or safflower instead of butter, lard, or shortening during cooking and at the table can help lower LDL.
- Apples, grapes, strawberries, and citrus fruits. These fruits are rich in pectin, a type of soluble fiber that lowers LDL.
- Soybeans. Consuming soybeans and foods made from soybeans, such as tofu and soy milk, was once touted as an effective way to lower cholesterol. Analyses show the effect is smaller, suggesting that consuming 25 grams of soy protein per day (10 ounces of tofu or 2 1/2 cups of soy milk) may lower LDL by 5%.
- Fatty Fish: Eating fish 2 to 3 times a week can lower LDL in two ways: by replacing meat, which contains LDL-raising saturated fats, and by consuming omega-3 fats, which lower LDL.[12]

---

[12] Harvard Health Publishing - https://www.health.harvard.edu/heart-health/11-foods-that-lower-cholesterol (Published in March 2024)

Not all cholesterol comes from the food we eat. About 80% of it is made in the **liver** in a complicated 37-step process. There are several things that can cause your cholesterol and triglycerides to rise: this could be because you eat a lot of saturated fats, don't exercise enough, have genetic conditions that don't process fats normally, or you could have another medical condition.
A simple cholesterol test and healthy changes to how you live can help most people keep their cholesterol values in a healthy range.

Blood pressure, the silent killer[13]

Blood pressure is how hard your blood is pushing against the artery walls.
During the day, your blood pressure usually goes up and down.
There are two numbers used to measure blood pressure. The first number, **systolic** blood pressure, shows how much pressure is in your vessels when your heart beats. The second number is **diastolic** blood pressure, and it shows the pressure when your heart is not beating.
Often systolic blood pressure (the first number) is seen as a major risk factor for heart disease in people over 50. In most people, systolic blood pressure slowly rises with age. This is because as people get older, their large arteries get stiffer, plaque builds up over time, and heart and vascular diseases become more common.
Less than 120 mmHg systolic and 80 mmHg diastolic is a healthy blood pressure reading.

---

[13] American Heart Association - https://www.heart.org/en/health-topics/high-blood-pressure/understanding-blood-pressure-readings (Reviewed in May 2023)

In the following table you can find healthy and unhealthy blood **pressure ranges**, as recommended by the American Heart Association.

BLOOD PRESSURE CATEGORY	**SYSTOLIC (mm Hg)**	**and/or**	**DIASTOLIC (mm Hg)**
Normal	Less than 120	and	Less than 80
Elevated	120 – 129	and	Less than 80
Hypertension stage 1	130 – 139	or	80 – 89
Hypertension stage 2	140 or higher	or	90 or higher
Hypertensive crisis (consult your doctor immediately)	Higher than 180	or	Higher than 120

People who already have elevated blood pressure are likely to get **hypertension** if they don't do something to control it. It is more likely that you will get heart disease, have a heart attack, or have a stroke if your blood pressure is high.

High blood pressure is called the "silent killer" because most people don't know they have it because they don't see any symptoms or feel any pain.

When you have high blood pressure, the pressure of the blood moving through your arteries slowly rises and it **may cause**[14]:

- **Damage and narrow vessels**. High blood pressure can hurt the cells that line the inside of the vessels. When fats from food get into the system, they can build up in arteries that are already damaged. Over time, the walls of arteries lose their elasticity, which makes it harder for blood to flow through the body.
- **Aneurysms**. Over time, the steady pressure of blood moving through an artery can make a part of its wall get bigger and form

[14] American Heart Association - https://www.heart.org/en/health-topics/high-blood-pressure/health-threats-from-high-blood-pressure (Reviewed in March 2022)

an aneurysm. An aneurysm could burst, causing internal bleeding that could be life-threatening. Any artery can get an aneurysm, but the aorta, which is the body's biggest artery, gets it most often.

- **Left heart to get bigger**. It takes more work for the heart to pump blood to all parts of the body when blood pressure is high. The lower left heart chamber (left ventricle) gets thicker because of this. Heart attack, heart failure, and sudden cardiac death are more likely to happen if this happens.
- **Heart failure**. In the long-term, high blood pressure can weaken the heart muscle and make it work less well because it puts so much stress on it. Eventually, the overwhelmed heart starts to fail.
- **Dementia**. Some types of dementia are caused by arteries that are narrowed or stopped, which cuts off blood flow to the brain. Vascular dementia can also be caused by a stroke that cuts off blood flow to the brain.
- **Kidney failure**. One of the main reasons people lose their kidneys is high blood pressure. Kidneys can't clear waste out of the blood properly when blood vessels are damaged, so dangerous amounts of fluid and waste build up. Dialysis or a kidney donation treat this organ failure.
- **Retinopathy** is the name for damage to the blood vessels in the eye. If the blood vessels in the retina (the light-sensitive tissue at the back of the eye) get hurt, it can bleed, blur your vision, or even make it impossible to see at all. Having both diabetes and high blood pressure makes you more likely to get retinopathy.
- Men who are 50 years or older are more likely to have **erectile dysfunction**, which means they can't get or keep an erection. But men with high blood pressure are even more likely to have trouble getting or keeping an erection, since high blood pressure can make it hard for blood to move to the penis. Women with high blood pressure may also have problems with their sex lives, because less blood flow to the vagina can make you less sexually aroused, making your vagina dry or hard to get an orgasm.

All about heart rate[15]

Knowing your heart rate can help you keep track of your fitness level and might even help you spot health problems before they get worse, even if you're not an athlete.

The number of times your heart beats every minute is your heart rate, also known as **pulse**. Different people have different values of normal heart rates. Being aware of yours can help you figure out how healthy your heart is.

The rate and consistency of your pulse can change as you get older. This could be a sign of a heart problem or another problem that needs to be treated.

It's very easy to **calculate** your pulse with a wearable fitness tracker, but you can also do it by hand if you don't have one. Your wrist, the inside of your elbow, the side of your neck, and the top of your foot are the best places to feel your pulse. Place your finger over your pulse and count how many times it beats in one minute. This will give you the most exact reading.

When you're not working out, your heart pumps the least amount of blood possible, which is called your **resting heart rate**. If you are sitting and calm, your heart rate should be between 60 and 100 beats per minute.

A heart rate lower than 60, on the other hand, doesn't always mean there is a problem. This is also true for people who are very athletic or who do a lot of physical exercise. A person's resting heart rate can be as low as 40 because their heart muscle is in better shape and doesn't have to work as hard to keep a steady beat. In this case, the resting pulse doesn't change much when you do a little or a lot of physical exercise.

---

[15] American Heart Association - https://www.heart.org/en/health-topics/high-blood-pressure/the-facts-about-high-blood-pressure/all-about-heart-rate-pulse (Reviewed in May 2023)

The average heartbeat of a woman is eight beats per minute faster than that of a man, because women have smaller hearts and they have to beat faster to pump the same amount of blood.
Tell your doctor if your pulse is very low or if you often have fast heart rates that you can't explain, especially if they make you feel weak, dizzy, or faint. Your doctor will decide if it's an emergency.

When you **work out**, whether you want to lose weight or just get the most out of your workout, this simple method will help you stay in the right training zone. Your goal heart rate helps you hit the mark, so every step, swing, and squat gives you the most benefit.
Your heart rate at its fastest is about 220 minus your age. The target heart rate for mild activity is between 50% and 70% of maximum heart rate, while for vigorous activity, it is between 70% and 85%.
If your heart rate is too high, you are pushing too much, so slow down! If your heart rate is too low and the level of energy feels "light" to "moderate," you might want to work out a little harder, especially if you're trying to lose weight.
When you first start, aim for the lower range of your goal zone (50 percent) and work your way up. Over time, you'll be able to work out at up to 85% of your maximum heart rate without feeling too tired.[16]

---

[16] American Heart Association - https://www.heart.org/en/healthy-living/fitness/fitness-basics/target-heart-rates (Reviewed in March 2021)

How to prevent CVDs

People who are behaviorally at risk may have high blood pressure, high blood sugar, high fat levels in the blood, and being overweight or obese.

- Cessation of **tobacco** use[17, 18]: There are chemicals in cigarette smoke that make the cells that line blood vessels swell and inflamed, and this can make the blood valves narrow, which can cause a lot of heart problems.
  The 2014 Surgeon General's Report on smoking and health says that smoking is a major cause of cardiovascular disease (CVD) and is responsible for about 1 in 4 deaths from CVD. Heart disease is 2 to 4 times more likely to happen to smokers than to people who don't smoke. People who smoke cigarettes are twice as likely to have a stroke. People who smoke less than 5 cigarettes a day may already have early signs of CVD, and the chance of getting CVD goes up with the number of cigarettes smoked every day and with long-term smoking. Heart disease is still more likely to happen even if you smoke cigarettes with less tar or nicotine. Also, people who don't smoke can get heart disease from being around people who smoke: about 34,000 nonsmokers die each year in the US from heart disease after being around people who smoke. Secondhand smoke is smoke that users breathe out, but also smoke from the end of a lit cigarette, cigar, or pipe is included.
- Reduction of **salt**[19]: A daily salt intake of 5 grams more (2000 mg of sodium) is linked to a 17% higher risk of all cardiovascular disease and, more importantly, a 23% higher risk of stroke.[20]

---

[17] Centers for Disease Control and Prevention - https://www.cdc.gov/tobacco/sgr/50th-anniversary/pdfs/fs_smoking_cvd_508.pdf (Accessed in May 2024)

[18] Johns Hopkins Medicine - https://www.hopkinsmedicine.org/health/conditions-and-diseases/smoking-and-cardiovascular-disease (Accessed in May 2024)

[19] American Heart Association - https://www.heart.org/en/healthy-living/healthy-eating/eat-smart/sodium/sodium-and-salt (Reviewed in December 2022)

When you have too much sodium in your blood, it pulls water into your blood vessels. This makes the volume of the blood inside them bigger. As a consequence, blood pressure goes up when more blood moves through your arteries. It's like turning up the water pressure in a yard hose: as more water flows through it, the pressure rises. Moreover, it takes more work for the heart to pump more blood through the body when blood flow goes up.
Some foods already have too much sodium even in them before we use the saltshaker at the table. More than 70% of the sodium we eat comes from ready-made, packed, and restaurant foods, because salt is added to foods to make them taste better, keep them fresh longer, and lower the risk of bacteria. The other 15% of sodium we eat comes from food itself, and the other 11% comes from salt added to food or to our plates. The Dietary Guidelines for Americans say that each day we should eat no more than 2,3 grams of salt, about 1 teaspoon.
Here are the top 10 foods that are high in sodium: breads, pizza, sandwiches, cold cuts, luncheon and salted meats, soups, burritos and tacos, savory snacks, chicken, cheese, and egg dishes.

- More **fruit** and **vegetables**[21]: In 2017, not eating enough fruits and vegetables was linked to an estimated 3.9 million deaths around the world.[22] A lot of fruits and veggies are high in vitamin C and beta-carotene, which is a type of vitamin A. These help stop or slow down atherosclerosis by reducing cholesterol and other substances from building up in the arteries. They do

---

[20] BMJ Journal - "Salt intake, stroke, and cardiovascular disease: meta-analysis of prospective studies" (Published in November 2009)
[21] Heart & Stroke - https://www.heartandstroke.ca/healthy-living/healthy-eating/vegetables-and-fruit (Accessed in May 2024)
[22] World Health Organization - https://www.who.int/tools/elena/interventions/fruit-vegetables-ncds (Updated in August 2023)

this by acting as antioxidants in your body. As an added bonus, most fruits and veggies are low in calories, fat, and salt.

- Regular **physical activity**[23]: Heart disease and stroke are 45% less likely to happen to runners. A daily exercise plan can help: it lowers blood pressure, lowers the chance of getting diabetes, keeps your weight at a healthy level, lessens inflammation all over the body, makes it easier for muscles to take oxygen out of the blood so the heart doesn't have to pump as much blood to them, lowers hormones that can put extra strain on the heart, slows down heart rate, boosts HDL ("good" cholesterol), and helps keep triglycerides in check.
- Avoiding harmful use of **alcohol**[24]: People have different ideas about whether or not drinking in moderation is good for your heart. The key word here is "moderate".

  A woman who drinks moderately has one drink a day, while a man should have no more than 1 or 2. A drink may not be as much as you think: 12 ounces (350 ml) of beer, 4 ounces (120 ml) of wine, or 1.5 ounces (45 ml) of 80-proof spirits.

  On the other hand, heavy drinking is linked to a number of health issues, such as heart problems. Too much drinking can cause high blood pressure and weight gain, providing an excess of calories.

  Some studies have found a link between drinking booze in moderation and a lower chance of dying from heart disease. But those studies don't make it easy to figure out cause and effect. It's possible that people who drink red wine have better incomes, which are linked to more education and easier access to healthier foods. In the same way, people who drink red wine may be more likely to eat a heart-healthy diet. If you drink a

---

[23] John Hopkins Medicine - https://www.hopkinsmedicine.org/health/wellness-and-prevention/exercise-and-the-heart (Accessed in May 2024)

[24] John Hopkins Medicine - https://www.hopkinsmedicine.org/health/wellness-and-prevention/alcohol-and-heart-health-separating-fact-from-fiction (Accessed in May 2024)

modest amount of alcohol, it may help to slightly raise your levels of "good" HDL cholesterol. Antioxidants found in red wine have also led researchers to think that it might be good for your heart.

- Decrease of **stress**: A joke a day may help keep the heart doctor away. Laughter can help heart health by lowering stress and relaxing blood vessels. Being happy can also make you less likely to get heart problems.
  A man's risk of dying from heart disease could be cut in half if he has an active sex life. One British study suggests that having an orgasm 3 or 4 times a week might make guys much less likely to have a heart attack or stroke. It's not clear if sex works better for women's hearts, but a healthy love life seems to mean a healthy body as a whole. Moreover, sexual activity is a great way to relieve stress and to work out—each half-hour burns about 85 calories.
- **Genetics, diabetes, gender** (men are more likely to get CVD younger than women), and **age** (the older you are, the more likely you are to get CVD) are some other factors.

Having a **pet** might make you healthier, happier, and less stressed. It may also lower your blood sugar, blood pressure, cholesterol, and weight. People who have dogs are more likely to do the suggested amount of exercise moving around with your pet, whether you're inside or outside. Dog owners are 34% more likely to walk at least 150 minutes a week.[25]

---

[25] American Heart Association - https://www.heart.org/en/healthy-living/healthy-bond-for-life-pets/pet-owners (Reviewed June 2022)

Recognize cardiovascular attacks[26]

A **heart attack** happens when a coronary artery that brings blood to the heart gets stopped so there is less oxygen getting to your heart muscle. This means that the longer the blockage is not handled, the more damage it does. If you don't get help right away to get the blood flowing again, the damage could be permanent or even deadly.
Symptoms of a heart attack include:

- Pain or discomfort in the center of the chest
- Pain or discomfort in the arms, the left shoulder, elbows, jaw, or back
- Difficulty in breathing
- Nausea or vomiting
- Light-headedness or faintness
- Cold sweat
- Turning pale

If you or someone you know is having heart attack symptoms for more than 10 minutes of rest, if the symptoms are severe, or if they are getting worse, you should get medical help right away.

Ischemic strokes happen when a blood clot blocks or plugs a blood vessel in the brain. Brain cells start to die in minutes, so the best stroke treatments can only be used if the stroke is found and identified within 3 hours of the first signs. If people who have had a stroke don't get to the hospital on time, they might not be eligible for these treatments.
People who have had an ischemic stroke often feel weak and numb in one side of their body, usually in their face, arm, or leg. Some other signs are sudden onset of:

- Confusion, difficulty speaking or understanding speech
- Difficulty seeing with one or both eyes
- Difficulty walking, dizziness and loss of balance or coordination
- Severe headache with no known cause

---

[26] Heart Foundation - https://www.heartfoundation.org.au/bundles/your-heart/heart-attack (Accessed in May 2024)

- Fainting or unconsciousness

Act **F.A.S.T.** to identify stroke![27]

If you think someone may be having a stroke, act F.A.S.T. and do the following test:

- F—Face: Ask the person to smile. Does one side of the face droop?
- A—Arms: Ask the person to raise both arms. Does one arm drift downward?
- S—Speech: Ask the person to repeat a simple phrase. Is the speech slurred or strange?
- T—Time: If you see any of these signs, call emergency right away.

Note the time when any symptoms first appear. This information helps health care providers determine the best treatment for each person.

[27] Centers for Disease Control and Prevention - https://www.cdc.gov/stroke/signs_symptoms.htm (Reviewed in May 2022)

The mystery around cancer[28]

The **word** "cancer" comes from the Latin word for "crab", since in the past doctors called some tumors that had lines or pieces that stuck out from the main body "crab-like" or "cancerous". The Edwin Smith Papyrus dated back to 1600 B.C., has the first written account of cancer, and it talks about how a tool called the fire drill was used to remove breast cancers.[29]

Every day, about 330 billion cells are replaced, which is about 1% of all the cells in our bodies. In other words, in 80 to 100 days, 30 trillion will have replenished, which is a new you. A healthy body, cells divide and grow to make more cells when needed. Cells die when they get old or damaged, and new cells grow in their place, however, some cells in the body **grow out of control** and spread to other places of the body, and this is what defines cancer.

When cancer gets into important systems like the liver, lungs, or brain and stops them from working right, it can kill you.

There are two possible causes of these problems: cancer that starts in an important system or cancer that has spread from one place to another. It gets harder to control cancer as it spreads to other parts of the body.

[28] National Cancer Institute - https://www.cancer.gov/about-cancer/understanding/what-is-cancer (Updated in October 2021)

[29] Roche - https://www.roche.com/stories/9-things-about-cancer (Accessed in May 2024)

Genetic changes that cause cancer can happen **because**:

- Of errors that occur as cells divide
- Of damage to DNA caused by harmful substances in the environment
- They were inherited from our parents

Cells with broken DNA are usually killed off by the body before they become cancerous, but as we age, our bodies become less able to do that. Part of the reason why cancer risk goes up with age is because of this.

People can't catch cancer from someone else, consequently things like kissing, hugging, sharing food, or breathing the same air cannot spread cancer. Cancer cells from one person can't live in the body of a healthy person, because the immune system looks for and kills alien cells, even cancer cells.

Even though **benign tumors** can be painful and even dangerous, they are not as dangerous as **malignant tumors**. Malignant cells are more likely to metastasize or spread to other parts of the body, while benign tumors don't usually attack and spread. The malignant also grows more quickly.

At first glance, it might seem clear that benign tumors are not dangerous and malignant tumors are, however, the lines between the two are not always clear. Yet it's very important to tell the difference between the two.[30]

Around the world, there were about 18.1 million cases of cancer in 2020. Because of this growing problem, preventing cancer is one of the most important public health issues of our time.

Around the world, 28 million people have survived cancer. Thank goodness, cancer doesn't always mean death, especially with all the progress made in the last few decades. Even though the number of

---

[30] Cancer Center - https://www.cancercenter.com/community/blog/2023/01/whats-the-difference-benign-vs-malignant-tumors (Published in January 2023)

people getting cancer is increasing, more people are beating it than ever before in many countries.[31]

Most common cancers[32]

Cancer is not just one disease. There are more than **200 different kinds** of cancer. Most of the time, the names come from the organs or tissues where the cancers start, but sometimes they come from the type of cell that made them. There are different types of cancer that grow at different speeds.

The most common cancers globally are listed in the tables below:

Rank	Cancer	New cases in 2020	% of all cancers	Rank men	Rank women
1	Breast	2,261,419	12.5		1
2	Lung	2,206,771	12.2	1	3
3	Colorectal	1,931,590	10.7	3	2
4	Prostate	1,414,259	7.8	2	
5	Stomach	1,089,103	6.0	4	7
6	Liver	905,677	5.0	5	9
7	Cervix uteri	604,127	3.3		4
8	Esophagus	604,100	3.3	7	13
9	Thyroid	586,202	3.2	16	5
10	Bladder	573,278	3.2	6	17

[31] Roche - https://www.roche.com/stories/9-things-about-cancer (Accessed in May 2024)
[32] World Cancer Research Fund - https://www.wcrf.org/cancer-trends/worldwide-cancer-data (Accessed in May 2024)

But **how many people die** of cancer each year? [33]
Around 10 million died from cancer in 2020 globally.
About 610.000 of them have been reported only in the United States in 2023, where lung and bronchus cancer killed the most people, 127.070, which are almost 3 times as many deaths from colon cancer, the second most common cause of cancer death.

Cancer type	**Deaths in US in 2023**
Lung and bronchus	127,070
Colon and rectum	52,550
Pancreas	50,250
Breast	43,700
Prostate	34,700
Liver and Intrahepatic Bile Duct	29,380
Leukemia	23,710
Non-Hodgkin Lymphoma	20,180

Most impactful cancers

Breast cancer[34]: The most common type of cancer in the world is breast cancer. Women are more likely than men to get breast cancer, but men can also get it (in the US, about 1 in 100 cases of breast cancer are found in men). There is some confusion about why the left breast is 5–10% more likely to get cancer than the right breast, as well as the left side of the body is also 10% more likely to get melanoma, a type of skin cancer.
There are different signs and symptoms of breast cancer in different people, while some people don't have any changes at all. Some warning signs of breast cancer are:

- Any change in the size or the shape of the breast, new lump, thickening or swelling

[33] National Cancer Institute - https://seer.cancer.gov/statfacts/html/common.html (Accessed in May 2024)
[34] Centers for Disease Control and Prevention - https://www.cdc.gov/cancer/breast/basic_info/what-is-breast-cancer.htm (Reviewed in July 2023)

- Irritation or dimpling of the breast skin, and redness/flaky skin or pulling in the nipple area
- Nipple discharge other than breast milk, including blood
- Pain in any area of the breast.

To reduce the risk of breast cancer:

- Ask your doctor about the risks related to hormone of replacement therapy or oral contraceptives and find out if they are right for you
- Breastfeed your children, if possible
- If you have a family history of breast cancer, talk to your doctor about other ways to lower your risk
- Ask your health care provider about the best ways to get screened. Screening for breast cancer can't stop people from getting it, but it can help find it early, when it's easier to treat.
  The US Preventive Services Task Force says that women between the ages of 50 and 74 who have an average chance of getting breast cancer should get a mammogram every 2 years. Women who are 40 to 49 years old should talk to their doctor or other health care provider about when to start and how often to get a mammogram.

So far, the best studies haven't found any proof that the chemicals in antiperspirants and deodorants are linked to changes in breast tissue.

Lung cancer[35]: The cancer that kills the most people is lung and bronchus cancer. Older people are more likely to get lung cancer: there are more than 4 in 10 people with lung cancer in the UK who are 75 years or older, and people younger than 40 rarely have it.
Lung cancer can happen to people who have never smoked, but smoking is the most common cause (more than 70% of cases). This is because people who smoke regularly breathe in a lot of harmful chemicals.

---

[35] National Health Service - https://www.nhs.uk/conditions/lung-cancer (Reviewed in November 2022)

In the early stages of lung cancer there are usually no signs or symptoms. Most of the time, you won't know you have lung cancer until it has spread to other parts of your body or through your lungs. This means that the prognosis is not as good as it is for many other types of cancer.

However, many people with the disease eventually develop symptoms such as a persistent cough, coughing up blood, constant shortness of breath, feeling tired all the time, losing weight, and having an ache or pain when they breathe or cough. If these things happen to you, you should see a doctor.

4 out of 10 people who are diagnosed with this condition live at least 1 year, and 1 out of 10 live at least 10 years.

Survival rates are very different based on how far the cancer has spread when it is found, so it can make a big difference if you catch it early.

Colorectal cancer[36] is based in the colon or rectum. It is also known as colon cancer for short. Abnormal growths, called polyps, can show up in the colon or rectum, and some of these polyps may turn into cancer over time. Polyps can be removed before they turn into cancer with the help of screening tests, when it is easiest to treat. In general, getting screened for colorectal cancer regularly starting at age 45 is the best way to lower your chance of getting it.

Pancreas[37]: The pancreas is a gland that looks like a thin pear 6 inches (15 centimeters) long lying on its side. Two main jobs of the pancreas are to make juices that help break down food and hormones, like insulin, that help keep blood sugar levels in check.

For several reasons, it's hard to find and diagnose pancreatic cancer: in its early stages, there are no obvious signs or symptoms; when they are

---

[36] Centers for Disease Control and Prevention - https://www.cdc.gov/cancer/colorectal/basic_info/what-is-colorectal-cancer.htm (Reviewed in February 2023)

[37] National Cancer Institute - https://www.cancer.gov/types/pancreatic/patient/pancreatic-treatment-pdq (Updated in May 2023)

present, the signs and symptoms of pancreatic cancer look like those of many other illnesses; and the pancreas is hidden behind other organs.

Prostate[38]: The main job of the prostate and seminal vesicles is to make fluid for semen. In its early stages, prostate cancer might not show any clear signs, so if any of these things happen, you should see a doctor:

- Frequent need to pass urine
- Trouble passing urine, pain, burning or weak urine flow
- Blood in the urine
- Painful ejaculation, or pain in the lower pelvic zone, lower back, hips, or upper thighs, or in the bones in general
- Loss of hunger or of weight

Skin[39-40]: Always check your skin. 1 in 5 Americans will get skin cancer at some point in their lives, making it the most common type of cancer in the U.S. A lot of people die every day from melanoma, the deadliest type of skin cancer. But skin cancer, including melanoma, is very easy to treat if it is found early. People with melanoma who are found and treated before it gets to the lymph nodes have a 98% chance of living for at least 5 years.

---

[38] Urology Care Foundation - https://www.urologyhealth.org/urologic-conditions/prostate-cancer (Updated in February 2023)

[39] American Academy of Dermatology Association - https://www.aad.org/public/everyday-care/skin-care-basics/care/skin-care-tips-dermatologists-use (Accessed in May 2024)

[40] Skin Cancer Foundation - https://www.skincancer.org/blog/surprising-danger-planes-trains-automobiles (Published in April 2021)

The UV Index tells us every day about how strong the UV rays will be in the US: https://enviro.epa.gov/envirofacts/uv/search

If the UV index in your area is 3 or higher, protect your skin from the sun as much as possible: stay in the shade and cover your arms and legs; cover your face, head, ears, and neck with a wide-brimmed hat; wear sunglasses that wrap around and block both UVA and UVB rays; use a broad range sunscreen with at least 15 SPF (Sun Protective Factor).[41]
You can find out if someone has melanoma by looking for the ABCDEs:

- A stands for ASYMMETRY: One half of the spot is unlike the other half.
- B stands for BORDER. The spot has an irregular, scalloped, or poorly defined border.
- C stands for COLOR. The spot has varying colors from one area to the next
- D stands for DIAMETER. While melanomas are usually greater than 6 mm, or about the size of a pencil eraser, when diagnosed, they can be smaller.
- E stands for EVOLVING. The spot looks different from the rest or is changing in size, shape, or color.

Record your spots, so you can regularly track changes.

[41] Centers for Disease Control and Prevention - https://www.cdc.gov/cancer/skin/basic_info/prevention.htm (Reviewed in April 2023)

Some common questions are:[42]

- Is indoor tanning ok?
  People who tan indoors are more likely to get skin cancer than people who smoke.
- Do people with dark skin get sunburnt?
  Dark or brown skinned people don't burn as quickly and are less likely to get skin cancer. But they can still get burned, though their skin might not change color but feel itchy or pink. Skin cancer can happen to anyone, no matter what color their skin is. To make vitamin D, we all need to be outside in the sun, but people with darker skin may be more likely to not get enough vitamin D because they need to be in the sun longer to produce it.
- Can UV rays be reflected?
  Up to 85% of UV rays are turned back into light by snow, 15% by sand, and 10% by water.
- Can you get sunburnt when it's cloudy?
  Clouds block some UV, but over 90% can still pass through light clouds and cause sunburn.
- Does glass block UV Rays?
  Glass does a good job of blocking UVB rays, but not UVA rays. Most side, back, and sunroof windows aren't cleaned to block UVA rays like windshields are, so keep yourself and your family safe from the sun when you're in your car. For long-term peace of mind, you might want to put clear UV-blocking window film in your car.
- Can skin cancer form on the lips?
  Yes, so make sure you put on lip balm or lipstick with sunscreen that has at least an SPF 30 rating before going outside. If your lips are cracked or dry, put on petroleum jelly to make them feel better.

[42] Cancer Research UK - https://www.cancerresearchuk.org/about-cancer/causes-of-cancer/sun-uv-and-cancer/the-uv-index-and-sunburn-risk (Reviewed in November 2023)

The 10 commandments of cancer prevention[43]

That's great that you get it diagnosed early, but can you do even better? Is there a way to avoid getting cancer in the first place? It is true, even though it sounds too good to be true. Scientists at the Harvard School of Public Health think that up to 75% of cancer deaths in the United States can be avoided. This means that globally 2.4 million to 3.7 million deaths could have been avoided every year, considering that over 80% of these deaths happen in low- and middle-income countries, and only 5%–10% of all cancers are completely passed down through families.

The 10 commandments of cancer prevention are:

1. Avoid **tobacco** in all its forms, including exposure to secondhand smoke. In the United States, smoking is the main reason people die prematurely and that could be avoided. There is no amount of smoking that is healthy. There are many chemicals in tobacco smoke that are bad for both users and people who don't smoke. Around 250 of the more than 7,000 chemicals found in tobacco smoke are known to be bad for you, and at least 69 of them can cause cancer. When people smoke, they may get cancer of the cervix, larynx (voice box), mouth, esophagus, throat, bladder, kidney, liver, stomach, pancreas, colon, rectum, as well as acute myeloid leukemia. Cancers of the mouth, stomach, and pancreas are more likely to happen to people who use smokeless tobacco like snuff or chewing tobacco.[44]
2. **Eat properly**. Cut down on red meat and saturated fats, which may raise your chance of colon cancer and a more aggressive form of prostate cancer. Some chemicals, like nitrates, have been added to processed meat to make it last longer or taste better. Ham, bacon, corned beef, and some sausages like salami,

---

[43] Harvard Health Publishing - https://www.health.harvard.edu/newsletter_article/the-10-commandments-of-cancer-prevention (Published in October 2019)

[44] National Cancer Institute - https://www.cancer.gov/about-cancer/causes-prevention/risk/tobacco/cessation-fact-sheet (Reviewed in December 2017)

chorizo, and hot dogs are all processed meats. Red meat is any kind of fresh, ground, or frozen beef, pork, or lamb. You are not more likely to get cancer if you eat white meat like chicken and fish. You might want to cut back on processed foods and red meat if you eat them most days. If you eat a lot of processed and red meat, the government says you should cut back to 70g or less per day: this is the same size as 3 ham slices, 2 bacon slices, or 1 small beef burger. If you eat less prepared foods and red meat, you are less likely to get cancer. This is true no matter how much you eat. Fruits, veggies, and whole grains should all be eaten more often.[45]

3. **Exercise** regularly. Being active (even if you don't lose weight) has been linked to a lower risk of getting breast, bowel, and colon cancer. Less estrogen and insulin in the body can circulate if you practice sports and at healthy weight: hormones like estrogen and insulin can make breast cells divide more often, which raises the chance of getting cancer. Additionally, your immune system will work better if you exercise and have a healthy weight. This is important also because the body will be able to find and kill cells that might turn into cancer better. Then, we can get rid of food faster through the bowel. That is, anything bad in the food we eat and the waste we make (poop) has less time to stay in our bowels. This might help keep you from getting bowel cancer. Finally, when you're active and at a good weight, inflammation goes down. When there is too much inflammation, our cells split more often, which raises the risk of getting cancer. [46]

---

[45] Cancer Research UK - https://www.cancerresearchuk.org/about-cancer/causes-of-cancer/diet-and-cancer/does-eating-processed-and-red-meat-cause-cancer (Reviewed in July 2023)

[46] Cancer Research UK - https://www.cancerresearchuk.org/about-cancer/causes-of-cancer/physical-activity-and-cancer/what-are-the-benefits-of-exercise (Reviewed in August 2023)

4. Stay **lean**. Being overweight or obese is the 2nd most common cause of cancer in the UK. 13 types of cancer are less likely to happen if you stay at a healthy weight. Breast and bowel cancer are two of the most common types of cancer in this group. Pancreatic, esophageal, and liver cancer are three of the hardest to treat. There's more going on inside your body than just extra fat: it sends information to other parts of your body, and these signs can tell our body's cells to grow more often, which can cause cancer. Immune cells go to places on the body where there are lots of fat cells, and inflammation can happen because of this, making cells grow faster. This can raise the chance of cancer over time. Sex hormone estrogen is made by fat cells after menopause. The risk of getting cancer goes up when this hormone makes cells in the breast and womb divide more often.[47]
5. If you choose to drink **alcohol**, limit yourself to an average of 1 drink a day. Too much alcohol raises the risk of cancer in the mouth, larynx (voice box), esophagus (food pipe), liver, stomach, and breast. Getting drunk can lead to cancer in many ways. Alcohol is changed into acetaldehyde in our bodies when we drink it, and acetaldehyde can damage our cells and can also stop cells from repairing this damage. Also, hormones like estrogen and insulin can rise in our bodies when we drink alcohol. Then, cells in the mouth and throat may be more likely to take in chemicals that are bad for them when you drink alcohol.

   Take note that even small amounts of booze are bad for your body, and it doesn't matter if you drink wine, beer, or liquor. Cancer can be caused by all kinds of drinking.[48]

---

[47] Cancer Research UK - https://www.cancerresearchuk.org/about-cancer/causes-of-cancer/bodyweight-and-cancer/how-does-obesity-cause-cancer (Reviewed in February 2023)

[48] Cancer Research UK - https://www.cancerresearchuk.org/about-cancer/causes-of-cancer/alcohol-and-cancer/how-does-alcohol-cause-cancer (Reviewed in September 2023)

6. Avoid unnecessary exposure to **radiation**
   Radon can raise the risk of getting lung cancer, so check your house for it.
   Don't worry about electromagnetic radiation from high-voltage power lines or radiofrequency radiation from microwaves and cell phones; they do not cause cancer.
   You should only get imaging tests when you really need them. CT scans and nuclear imaging, which need higher radiation doses than regular x-rays, are mostly to blame for the higher exposure in the US.[49]

Radiation exposure (in millisievert, mSv)	Medical imaging technique
22.7	Positron Emission Tomography — Computed Tomography (PET/CT): Whole body
8.7	Coronary Computed Tomography Angiography (CTA)
6	Computed Tomography (CT): Chest or Colonography
1.5	Computed Tomography (CT): Head and Neck, Brain, or Lung Cancer Screening
0.24	Screening Digital Mammography or 3D Mammogram
0.1	Chest X-Ray
0.005	Dental X-ray
0.001	Bone Densitometry (DEXA)
0	Ultrasound / Echography
0	Magnetic Resonance Imaging (MRI)

[49] American College of Radiology - https://www.acr.org/-/media/ACR/Files/Radiology-Safety/Radiation-Safety/Dose-Reference-Card.pdf (Published in May 2022)

The actual dose can be very different based on the size of the person and how the imaging is done. Also, keep in mind that because kids are of different sizes, the amounts given to them will be very different from those given to adults.
Ask your doctor if there is a lower-dose x-ray or a test that doesn't use radiation that could be used instead of the CT or nuclear medicine scan. For example, if ultrasound (which uses high-frequency sound waves) or MRI (which uses magnetic energy) could be used instead.
Unless you were exposed to high amounts of radiation when you were younger and were being treated for cancer, medical radiation doesn't seem to raise your risk of getting cancer very much. But we can't be sure because the damage from radiation usually takes a long time to show up, and the use of high-dose imaging has only grown since 1980. Because of this, you should stay away from medical radiation as much as possible until we know more. Several things can help you do that: discuss with your doctor about any high-dose diagnostic imaging; keep track of your x-ray history; think about getting a lower-dose radiation test; think about getting tests less often; and don't look for scans.[50]

7. Stay away from benzene, asbestos fibers, aromatic amines, and polychlorinated biphenyls (PCBs), as well as other **industrial and natural toxins**.
   In a technical sense, Teflon doesn't pose any health risks. As per the American Cancer Society (ACS), there are no proven risks to humans from using cookware coated with Teflon (or other non-stick surfaces). The chemical perfluorooctanoic acid (PFOA),

[50] Harvard Health Publishing - https://www.health.harvard.edu/cancer/radiation-risk-from-medical-imaging (Published in September 2021)

which has been used to make Teflon in the past, is thought to be bad for your health by some experts.[51]
The Food and Drug Administration (FDA) looked at many safety studies on each artificial sweetener to see if they could be harmful to people's health. The studies found no proof that these sweeteners cause cancer or other problems in people.

8. Avoid **infections** that contribute to cancer, including hepatitis viruses, HIV, and the human papillomavirus. A lot of them are spread sexually or through contaminated needles. About 15% to 20% of cancers in the world are linked infections. The United States and other developed countries have smaller rates than this, but it is even higher in developing countries. One reason for this is that some infections are more common in developing countries, and also because some factors that put people at risk for cancer, like being overweight, are more common in developed countries. There are different ways that infections can make someone more likely to get cancer. As an example, some viruses change the genes inside cells that decide how much they grow. These viruses can get into cells and add their own genes, which makes the cells grow out of control. Some diseases can make an area of the body inflamed for a long time, and this can cause changes in the immune cells close and in the cells that are nearby. Some infections can weaken the immune system as well, which usually helps keep the body safe from some cancers.[52]
9. Make quality **sleep** a priority. There isn't a lot of strong proof that sleep is linked to cancer, but not getting enough sleep is linked to weight gain, which is another risk factor.

---

[51] Cancer Center - https://www.cancercenter.com/community/blog/2021/09/does-teflon-cause-cancer (Published in September 2021)

[52] American Cancer Society - https://www.cancer.org/cancer/risk-prevention/infections/infections-that-can-lead-to-cancer/intro.html (Revised in July 2016)

10. Get enough **vitamin D**. There is some evidence that vitamin D may help lower the chance of prostate, colon, and other cancers, but this is still not proven. Everybody needs a different amount of sunshine to make vitamin D, so the time of day or year and the type of skin you have all play a role. People whose skin is lighter and more likely to burn should only be able to spend minutes in the sun without any protection. You might need more time to make enough vitamin D if you have darker skin. Most people should be able to get all the vitamin D they need from sunlight from late March or early April to the end of September. But from October to early March, the sun doesn't give us enough vitamin D. Many experts now say that people should get 800 to 1,000 IU of vitamin D every day. This is a goal that's hard to reach without taking a supplement, since foods like oily fish, red meat, liver, and egg whites don't contain enough vitamin D on their own.

    Don't count on other supplements, though.

Your mind

"Mens sana in corpore sano" - Juvenal (Roman poet, 2nd century AD)

"**A** healthy **mind** in a healthy **body**" is what this Latin saying means.
After more than 2 millennia, we are still arguing about this dualism, trying to figure out the parts of the biopsychosocial model of illness, and trying to make the sciences of the mind and biomedicine equal in terms of importance. We are slowly figuring out how mental and physical health are connected and how illnesses affect both.
WHO says that health is more than just not being sick or hurt. It's a state of full physical, mental, and social well-being.

Mental health is the state of being mentally well that lets people deal with life's stresses, see what they're capable of, learn and work well, and contribute to their community. As an important part of health and well-being, it supports our individual and group abilities to make choices, form connections, and change the world we live in. Everyone has the

right to good mental health, and it is very important for growth in the individual, the group, and the economy.
Mental health isn't just not having any mental illnesses. There is a complicated continuum that people experience in different ways, with varied levels of distress and difficulty and possible very different social and clinical outcomes.
Mental health conditions include mental disorders, psychosocial disabilities, and other mental states that cause a lot of distress, make it hard to do things, or put you at risk of hurting yourself.

Throughout our lives, many personal, social, and structural **factors** can work together to improve or worsen our mental health and move us up or down the mental health spectrum. Some psychological and biological traits, like emotional kills, drug use, and genetics, can make people more vulnerable to mental health problems. People are also more likely to get mental health problems if they are exposed to bad social, economic, geopolitical, and environmental situations, such as poverty, violence, inequality, and lack of resources for the environment.
You can face risks at any point in your life, but the ones that happen during developmentally sensitive times, like early childhood, are especially bad. For instance, it is known that harsh parenting and physical penalties are bad for kids' health, and bullying is a major cause of mental health problems.
Protective factors also show up at different times in our lives and help us be stronger. They include things like having good relationships with other people, getting a good education, having a good job, living in a safe area, and having a strong community.
On different levels, society has both things that can hurt and things that can help mental health. People, families, and groups are more likely to be hurt by local threats. Global threats, such as economic downturns, disease outbreaks, humanitarian crises, forced migration, and the worsening climate crisis, make everyone more at risk.
Each risk and protective factor can only tell you so few about the future. Many people who are exposed to a risk factor still don't get a mental health condition, and many people who are not exposed to a known risk

factor still get a mental health condition. In any case, the combining factors that affect mental health can either improve or worsen mental health.[53]

Complexity of the brain

One of the most complicated things in the world is the brain, so let’s first know it better, discovering some amazing things about your brain that will blow your mind.

A softball-sized group of cells, chemicals, and connective tissue make it up on one level, but on another, it's everything.

Brains feel like a treat made of loose gelatin, but brains that are taken out for research are treated in a special way to make them hard.

Your brain has about 100 billion neurons, which is about the same as there are stars in the Milky Way sky.

There are different kinds of brain cells, and they are all different sizes and shapes, and they do different things. Another thing is that you have at least as many glia cells as neurons, and they support, and help keep neurons from getting hurt. They also play key parts in how neurons talk to each other.

There are no pain sensors in the brain, so it can only feel good things. The meninges, which cover the brain, are where migraine and headache pain starts.

The brain is always changing as a result of what it learns, and this is called **neuroplasticity**. One of the most important things about the brain is that it can change and adapt to new situations. Neurons can change their strength, which is similar to how you can change the volume of a talk, on how they are linked to hundreds or thousands of other neurons by synapses, which are like links between neurons. Feel like your nerves can send signals as fast as Formula 1 cars (about 100 m/s or 360 km/h). Some parts of the brain can make brand-new neurons, and new

---

[53] World Health Organization - https://www.who.int/news-room/fact-sheets/detail/mental-health-strengthening-our-response (Published in June 2022)

connections can show up or go away. It is known that the brain can make new connections at any point in time.
Neurons can't talk to each other without these messages, which are known as action potentials. The Nobel Prize in 1963 was given for work that helped scientists figure out how action potentials are made.
Throughout our lives, our brains keep making new neurons, but there are only certain parts where this process called neurogenesis takes place: some examples are the striatum, which helps with movement and processing rewards, and the hippocampus, which is a key part of memory.

We don't just use 10% of our brains. Every part of our brain is used, though some are busier than others at any given time. It uses 20% of our energy, even though it only makes up 3% of our body weight, making it the most **energy-intensive** part of our bodies. But still, your brain uses only 20 watts of power, as a light bulb, which is very little. To understand better this efficiency, to mimic the brain's 100 trillion connections in real time, a computer would need 12 gigawatts, which is about 600 million times as much power!
The brain is consequently the "hottest" part of the body, being 2.5 degrees Celsius (4.5 degrees Fahrenheit) warmer than the rest of the body.[54, 55]

Stigma around mental illness[56]

More than half of people who have a mental problem don't get any **help** for it. People often don't get help or delay it because they're afraid of being treated differently or losing their jobs and way of life. In part, this

[54] Cleveland Clinic - https://health.clevelandclinic.org/brain-teasers-infographic (Published in December 2020)
[55] Queensland Brain Institute - https://qbi.uq.edu.au/10-amazing-facts-about-brain (Accessed in May 2024)
[56] American Psychiatric Organization - https://www.psychiatry.org/patients-families/stigma-and-discrimination (Reviewed in March 2024)

is because shame, bias, and discrimination against people with mental illness are still big issues.

Stigma against people with mental illness can be very clear or very subtle, but it can hurt them either way. There are many ways that people with mental illness are left out and treated against, but knowing what that looks like and how to stop it can help.
Stigma is often **caused** by not knowing or being afraid, moreover media portrayals of mental illness that are inaccurate or false add to both of these problems. A review of studies on stigma shows that while the public may accept the medical or genetic nature of a mental health disorder and the need for treatment, many people still have a negative view of those with mental illness.
Researchers identified several types of stigma, including: public stigma is when people don't like or accept people with mental illness; self-stigma is when people with mental illness don't like or accept their own condition, including feeling ashamed of it; and institutional stigma is when government and private organizations have rules that make it harder for people with mental illness to do things, whether they mean to or not. Some examples are not enough funding for studies into mental illness or not enough mental health services compared to other types of health care.

Stigma **affects** not only the person who has a mental illness but also the people who care about and support them, often family members.
Stigma about mental illness is especially a big problem in some racial and ethnic communities, and it can make it hard for people from those groups to get mental health treatments. For instance, in some Asian countries, getting professional help for a mental illness might go against the values of having a strong family, controlling your emotions, and not wanting to feel shame.

There are things that each of us can do to help **lessen the stigma** of mental illness, according to the National Alliance on Mental Illness (NAMI):

- Know or talk to someone who has a mental illness. When we know someone who has a mental illness, it makes it less scary and more real.
- Be transparent about your mental health, like by posting on social media. People who speak out and share their stories can make a difference.
- Learn more about the subject and share facts and experiences when someone says something bad or wrong.
- Be aware of the words you use and remind people that they matter.
- Draw comparison about how they would treat someone with cancer or diabetes to show that mental illness is similar to physical illness.
- Have compassion for people who are mentally ill.
- Be honest about treatment; make mental health care treatment normal, just like other types of health care treatment.
- Tell the media when they use stigmatizing language or tell stories about mental illness in a way that makes people feel bad about themselves.
- Choose to be strong instead of ashamed: "I fight stigma by choosing to live an empowered life. To me, that means owning my life and my story and refusing to allow others to dictate how I view myself or how I feel about myself". – Val Fletcher, long-time executive director of the Institute for Human Centered Design.

Alzheimer and other dementias[57]

Dementia is not a specific disease, but it is rather a general term for not being able to remember things, think clearly, or make choices, which makes it hard to do normal things. Dementia is not a normal part of getting older, even though it mostly happens to older people. Alzheimer's and other types of dementia kill 65% of women around the world, which is more than any other disease.

The **signs** of dementia can be very different from one person to the next because dementia is a broad word. Memory, attention, communication, reasoning, judgment, problem-solving, and visual perception are just a few of the things that people with dementia have trouble with.
Getting lost in a known area, using strange words to talk about everyday things, when you forget the name of a close friend or family member, forgetting about the past, or not being able to do things on your own, are signs that someone may have dementia.

In all cases of neurological dementia, like Alzheimer's, frontotemporal dementia, or Lewy body dementia, the disease starts in a certain part of the brain. After killing cells, they slowly spread to nearby areas.
For example, Alzheimer's starts in the hippocampus, which is often linked to memory. Over time, that harmful activity spreads to nearby memory stores and the frontal cortex, where it starts to change behavior and the way decisions are made. In its **last stages**, Alzheimer gets deep into the brain. This could stop basic body processes like breathing and heart rate.
In the past, complications like lung or urinary tract infections and falls have been the main reason people died as dementia got worse.[58]

---

[57] Centers for Disease Control and Prevention - https://www.cdc.gov/aging/dementia/index.html (Reviewed in April 2019)
[58] Columbia University - https://www.neurology.columbia.edu/news/understanding-how-dementia-causes-death-0 (Published in February 2023)

Most cases of dementia are caused by **Alzheimer**'s disease, which accounts for 60% to 80% of all cases. The main sign of the disease is having trouble remembering recent events, like a talk that happened minutes or hours ago. Later on, it gets harder to remember things that happened a long time ago. Then, other worries like having trouble walking or talking or behavioral changes also show up.
Most of the risk comes from family background. If you have a first-degree cousin with Alzheimer's disease, your chance of getting it goes up by 10% to 30%.

Even though getting older is the main factor that makes you more likely to get dementia, there are things you can do to **lower your own risk**:

- Regular physical activity: One of the best ways to lower your chance of dementia. It is good for your heart, blood flow, weight, and mental health.
- Choosing healthy foods: There is no one food, ingredient, or vitamin that can improve brain health on its own. What makes a difference is eating a variety of things in the right amounts.
- Don't smoke. If you smoke, you have a much greater chance of getting dementia later in life.
- Don't drink so much
- Keep your mind and social life active. Mental or social tasks may help your brain deal with illness better, relieve stress, and make you feel better. Anything that keeps your mind active, helps you process knowledge, and improves your thinking skills is good for your brain and lowers your risk. You might like apps that can keep your mind active, such as puzzles, memory, and board games. Conversations can also help you improve many mental skills, such as the ability to actively listen and communicate with another person, as well as the ability to think about what they are saying and how they feel.

Mental disorders[59]

A mental disorder is when a person's thinking, feeling, or acting is messed up in a way that is clinically significant. In most cases, it's linked to distress or problems in key areas of working, but mental disorders come in a lot of different forms. Still, there is effective psychological treatment available, and based on the age and severity, medication may be considered.

A lot of different personal, family, community, and structural **factors** can work together to help or hurt mental health at any given time. Even though most people are resilient, those who are subject to bad things like poverty, violence, disability, and unfairness are more likely to be affected. Some of the psychological and biological factors that can protect or put someone at risk are genetics and social skills. Many of the risk and protection factors are affected by changes in the way the brain works and is structured.

There were **970 million people** dealing with a mental disorder around the world in 2019. The most common ones were anxiety and depression, and the COVID-19 pandemic caused a big rise in the number of people living with them in 2020. Anxiety disorders and major depression disorders have both gone up by 26% and 28%, respectively, in just one year.

At the end of 2019, 301 million people, including 58 million kids and teens, had an **anxiety** condition. Anxiety disorders are marked by excessive fear and worry, along with changes in behavior that go along with them. There are serious enough symptoms to cause a lot of distress or make it hard to do things. To name a few, generalized anxiety disorder (which is marked by excessive worry), panic disorder (which is marked by panic attacks), social anxiety disorder (which is marked in social situations), and separation anxiety disorder (which is marked by

[59] World Health Organization - https://www.who.int/news-room/fact-sheets/detail/mental-disorders (Published in June 2022)

excessive fear about being away from people with whom the person has a close emotional connection).

More than 280 million people, including 23 million kids and teens, were **depressed** in 2019. Mood swings and short-lived emotional reactions to problems in daily life are not the same thing as depression. A person has a depressive episode when they feel sad, restless, or empty for most of the day, losing pleasure or interest in doing things, almost every day for at least 2 weeks. Along with these symptoms, the person may have trouble focusing, feel too guilty or not being good enough about themselves, lose hope about the future, think about suicide or dying, have trouble sleeping, lose or gain weight, or feel very tired or lacking energy.

Health and happiness go hand in hand[60]

Happiness is defined as the overall **appreciation** of one's life-as-a-whole, in short, how much one likes the life one lives.

People who describe themselves as happy tend to have fewer health problems, a lower risk of depression, and longer lives. Mind-body connection goes deeper than many people realize, and a troubled mind can contribute to health problems.

Several possible mechanisms are mentioned in the literature. The most commonly mentioned direct effect is that chronic unhappiness activates the fight-flight response, which is known to involve harmful effects in the long run, such as higher blood pressure and a lower immune response. The effect of negative mental states is well documented in psychosomatic medicine. Another commonly mentioned mechanism is better health behavior. Happy people are more inclined to watch their weight, are more perceptive of symptoms of illness and cope better with threatening information. Happy people also live healthier, they engage

[60] Harvard Health Publishing - https://www.health.harvard.edu/mind-and-mood/health-and-happiness-go-hand-in-hand (Published in November 2021)

more often in sports, and they tend to be more moderate with smoking and drinking.[61]

What if, though, you're not naturally happy? **How can you make yourself happy**, especially when things are hard?
It turns out that most people can make themselves happier. Some research shows that genetics determines about 50% of a person's overall happiness, 40% is up to people, and the last 10% relies on the situation.
In other words, even if you don't think you're happy, you probably have the power to change that.
That being said, even the happiest person finds it hard to stay positive all the time. Like any other part of health, happiness is a constant work in progress. But no matter how happy you are right now, there are things you can do to improve your mood and your physical and mental health. Here are some ideas you could use.

- **Keep in touch**. Strong ties with family and friends were found to be linked to happiness in a Harvard study.
- **Put up your hand**. Volunteering makes you feel good and gives you a sense of meaning. A 2016 study in BMJ found that the effect was strongest in people over the age of 70.
- **Do nice things for other people**. Choose a day and make it a point to do nice things for other people that you normally wouldn't. Being intentional about doing good things for other people can have positive benefits on your own health, even if it takes a lot of planning ahead of time.
- **Find your inner child**. You can do the things that made you happy as a child or young adult again when you get older. When you were younger, what made you happy? Get back into the games, sports, hobbies, or other things you liked when you were younger.

---

[61] Journal of Happiness Studies - https://link.springer.com/article/10.1007/s10902-006-9042-1 (Published in February 2007)

- **Get more time**. According to a study published in 2017 in the Proceedings of the National Academy of Sciences, people are happier with their lives when they spend their money on things that save them time, like getting someone else to do their chores, instead of things that they want. No matter how much money someone had, the result was the same.
- **Spend money on experiences**. Living a full life is another way that money can buy happiness. It also doesn't have to be an expensive trip. You could choose to eat dinner at a foreign restaurant, see a theater play in the afternoon, or go to an art show. Some studies show that people who spend money on experiences are happy in the long run because they make them remember good times, while on the other hand, buying things usually only brings short-term happiness.
- **Spend time with people who are happy**. Happiness can be contagious even through social networks. Your positive mood can start a chain effect where your contacts feel better being around you, who then make their contacts feel better, and so on. Also, the experts found that sadness doesn't spread as quickly as happiness does.
- **Look for greener**. EPJ Data Science released an online study in 2021 that looked at green spaces in 90 cities around the world and how they affected the people who lived there. No matter what the country's economy was like, it was found that people were happier when there was more urban green space around them, like parks, gardens, and riverbanks. Making your own green place can do the same thing, since a different study found that gardening at home can help your mental health in a way like how bike riding and walking can.
- **Change your habits**. A study that came out online in 2020 in Nature Neuroscience found that people are happier when their daily habits are more varied. Changes of any size can make a big difference. The results showed that changing your normal routine can make your life more interesting. For example, you

could try a new exercise plan every two weeks, listen to music instead of podcasts some days, or just take a different route to the store.

- **Take a moment to be thankful**. Make time to write down the things you're thankful for. Something you usually take for granted, like a house over your head and a family that cares about you, or something simple, like a compliment from someone you care about, a book you enjoy, the nice weather today, or a meal you had yesterday that tasted great.
- **Choose less often**. Researchers have found that when people have more choices, they are more likely to regret them and worry. It's easy to make choices that will keep you happy with a simple plan. When making a choice that won't have big effects, try giving yourself less time to think about it or picking from fewer options. Then, when you make a choice, don't change your mind about it. Think deeply about more important problems when you need to.

Suicide reality[62]

Every year, more than 700,000 people kill themselves, and every time someone kills themselves, many more try to do the same.

Suicide is the 4th **leading cause of death** among 15–29-year-olds, and 77% of suicides around the world happen in countries with low or middle wealth. About 20% of suicides around the world are thought to be caused by pesticide poisoning, but hanging and using a gun are also two other popular ways to kill yourself.

WHO's method to **preventing suicide** includes the following key interventions that have been shown to work:

- Make it harder for people to get suicide tools like pesticides, guns, and some medications
- Work with the media to make sure suicide stories are reported in a responsible way

[62] World Health Organization - https://www.who.int/news-room/fact-sheets/detail/suicide (Published in August 2023)

- Teach teens social and emotional life skills
- Find, evaluate, manage, and follow up with anyone who is showing signs of suicidal behavior as soon as possible

It is because of **stigma** that many people who are thinking about or have tried to kill themselves don't get the help they need. This is especially true when it comes to mental illnesses and suicide. People don't know that suicide is a big public health problem, and it's considered a taboo to talk about it in many places. This means that suicide prevention hasn't been given enough attention. As of now, only 38 countries globally say they have a national suicide prevention plan, and only a few countries have made suicide prevention a part of their health strategy.
To make success in preventing suicide, we need to break down social taboos and make people more aware of the problem.

Stress management[63-64]

"Fight or flight" is another name for the stress reaction. It's what the body does to get ready for or avoid danger. The stress reaction helps us deal with many problems when it is activated in the right way. Of course, things go wrong when this reaction is constantly sparked by everyday things like money problems, traffic jams, job worries, or relationship issues.

This can lead to **health problems**. One great example is having high blood pressure, which makes you more likely to get heart disease. The stress reaction also weakens the immune system, making people more likely to get colds and other illnesses. Stress that builds up can also make anxiety and sadness worse.

---

[63] Harvard Health Publishing - https://www.health.harvard.edu/mind-and-mood/relaxation-techniques-breath-control-helps-quell-errant-stress-response (Published in July 2020)
[64] Centers for Disease Control and Prevention - https://www.cdc.gov/mentalhealth/cope-with-stress/index.html (Reviewed in April 2023)

These things can happen because of stress:

- Feelings of fear, anger, sadness, worry, numbness, or frustration.
- Changes in appetite, energy, desires, and interests.
- Trouble concentrating and making decisions.
- Nightmares or problems sleeping.
- Physical reactions, such as headaches, body pains, stomach problems, or skin rashes.
- Worsening of chronic health problems and mental health conditions.
- Increased use of alcohol, illegal drugs (like heroin, cocaine, or methamphetamine), and misuse of prescription drugs (like opioids).

We wouldn't want to, but we can't stay away from everything that causes us stress. We can, however, learn better ways to deal with them. Inducing the **relaxation response** is one way. Cardiologist Dr. Herbert Benson came up with this method in the 1970s at Harvard Medical School. The relaxation response is a deep state of relaxation that can be triggered by a number of things, such as progressive muscle relaxation, yoga, meditation, and so on.

You can **deal with stress**, anxiety, grief, or fear in these ways:

- Take breaks from reading news stories, even ones on social media. Knowing about bad things happening all the time can be upsetting, but it's good to know about them. You might want to limit how often you check the news and take a break from your phone, TV, and computer screens for a while.
- Take good care of your body: Emotional health can be improved by taking care of your body.
- Drink less booze. Either don't drink at all or drink less. Men should have no more than two drinks a day, and women should have no more than one.

- Don't use illegal drugs or medicinal drugs in ways that aren't what the doctor told you to take. There is support for people who use drugs, and the first step to healing is to ask for help.
- Don't smoke, vape, or use any other nicotine products.
- Keep your normal checkups, tests, screenings, and shots with your doctor.
- Take some time to relax. Do something you enjoy, like take some deep breaths, stretch, or breathe.
- Talk to other people. Talk about your worries and how you feel with people you trust.

Be mindful[65]

It can be hard to pay attention to what's going on right now. A lot of the time, we think about what's going to happen next, or about things that happened in the past that we can't change. We might **miss the chance to live in the present**.

You can train yourself to pay attention to the present. Things like your ideas, feelings, sensations, and the world around you become clearer to you. You watch these moments without judging them. Mindfulness is the word for this.

Meditation in Buddhism is where mindfulness got its start. The goal of meditation is to make you more aware of your thoughts and help you focus.

Mindfulness is a word that most people have heard these days. There are now a lot of mindfulness programs in hospitals, schools, and businesses.

Studies show that focusing on the present moment can be **good for your health** and happiness.

For example, mindfulness-based therapies have been shown to help people who are depressed and anxious, moreover it has been shown to

[65] National Institutes of Health - https://newsinhealth.nih.gov/2021/06/mindfulness-your-health (Published in June 2021)

lower blood pressure and help people sleep better. It might even help people handle pain.
When you have depression, your thoughts can wander to the past or the future, and you may spend a lot of time thinking about bad things that happened in the past or worried about what will happen in the future.

A **sitting meditation** that is done in a quiet place can be part of mindfulness. You focus on your breathing or how your body feels during this exercise. You try to bring your mind back to the present moment when it wanders, like when you have thoughts about things you need to do.
Mindfulness doesn't need to be done while sitting still or in silence, though. Practice can be a part of everyday things you do, like eating or walking. You can also be aware when you're with other people.

It takes work **to become more mindful**, and here there are some ideas:

- Take a few deep breaths. Count to 4 as you breathe in through your nose, hold your breath for 1 second, and then breathe out through your mouth for 5 counts. Do it over and over.
- Take a walk. Pay attention to your breath and the sounds and things around you as you walk. If worries and thoughts come up, note them but then come back to the moment.
- Learn to eat with awareness. Pay attention to how each bite tastes, feels, and smells. Pay attention when your body says it's full or hungry.
- Look over your body. Pay close attention to how every part of your body feels. This might help you feel more in touch with your body.
- Look for tools on mindfulness, such as online programs and practices led by a teacher. A lot of tools and apps can be found online, but not all of them are the same. Medical schools and universities are good places to look for tools by experts, so check if they are based on facts.

Breath well

As babies, we come into the world by breathing in. We breathe out when we leave. In many languages, the word "exhale" means the same thing as "die". Because breathing is so important to life, it's not surprising that people have known for a long time that they need to control it to be healthier and more alive.
Most of the time, we don't even realize that we're breathing, but every day, we breathe about 22,000 times.
Breathing gives us power. Our lungs give us oxygen, which is the gas that keeps our bodies alive. When we take in air, our lungs remove oxygen and send it through our bloodstream to the organs and tissues that help us move, talk, and walk.
You can't breathe and swallow at the same time. This may seem like a no-brainer, but it's actually a protective evolutionary mechanism that keeps you from choking on your own food or even spit by mistake.
We normally breathe alternatively through one nostril and then the other, we just aren't aware of it. This keeps the air we breathe moist, so it doesn't irritate our lungs. However, our bodies rest one nose while the other works.

Your right and left **lungs** are not the same. There are 2 parts to the lung on the left side of your body, and there are 3 parts to the lung on your right side. Also, the left lung is about 10% smaller, which makes room for the heart.
You can live with only one lung, you can't do as much, but that doesn't mean you can't live a pretty normal life.
In your lungs about 2,400 kilometers of passageways are found, and there are also about 600 million air pockets called alveoli.[66]

Chinese Taoism and Hinduism both talked about a **"vital principle"** that runs through the body, like an energy or internal breath, as early as the first millennium B.C. They saw breathing as one of its forms. This force is

---

[66] Canadian Lung Association - https://www.lung.ca/lung-health/lung-info/breathing (Accessed in May 2024)

known as qi in Chinese and prana in Hinduism, one of the main concepts in yoga.
In fact, every method of meditation, rest, or calming down depends on breathing, which may be the thing that all of these methods have in common. Basic physiological research and studies on the effects of breath-control techniques support the idea that we should be aware of and manage our breathing.
Even a basic knowledge of how the body works can help you understand why controlled breathing can help you relax.

Everyone knows that how we **feel** has an effect on our bodies. You can tell when you're happy because the corners of your mouth turn up and the edges of your eyes wrinkle up in a certain way. In the same way, your breathing slows down and deepens when you feel safe and calm, when you are at rest, or when you are having a nice conversation. The parasympathetic nervous system is impacting your body and making you feel calm. On the other hand, your breathing speeds up and shallows down when you are scared, in pain, or tense and uncomfortable. Now the sympathetic nerve system is working, which controls how the body responds to stress in different ways. Not as many people know that the effects can also go the other way: the state of the body can change feelings. Research has shown that when your face smiles, your brain responds by making you feel better. Breathing in particular can change the way you think. Overall, studies show that these techniques help lower anxiety, but the anxiety doesn't go away totally. Being able to breathe better is a tool, not a cure-all. Clinical studies have shown that some methods work, but not all of them.[67]

Just like aerobic exercise makes your heart work better and your muscles stronger, **breathing exercises** can make your lungs work better. It's normal and easy to breathe when your lungs are healthy. If you work out regularly, you can make your lungs bigger, and people with big lungs

---

[67] Scientific American - https://www.scientificamerican.com/article/proper-breathing-brings-better-health (Published in January 2019)

can move air around their bodies more quickly. When you breathe in and out, a muscle called diaphragm does about 80% of the work to fill your lungs with oxygen and other gases and then empty them of waste gas.

Breath focus is a part of many methods that make you feel calm, and to start, you need to learn how to breathe deeply. Deep breathing is also known as abdominal, belly, diaphragmatic, and paced breathing. When you take a deep breath, the air that comes in through your nose fills your lungs all the way, and the lower belly rises.

A lot of us find it strange to breathe deeply. That's because of a number of things. For starters, body image issues make it harder in our society, since people tend to hold their stomach muscles in because they think a flat stomach looks good. This gets in the way of deep breathing and makes shallow breathing (called "chest breathing") seem normal, which increases tension and anxiety. The diaphragm can't move as far when you breathe shallowly, and the part of the lungs at the bottom doesn't get enough fresh air. That might make you stressed out and short of breath. Deep belly breathing helps with full oxygen exchange, which is the healthy exchange of oxygen entering the body for carbon dioxide leaving it. It's no surprise that it can slow the heartbeat and drop or keep blood pressure stable.

Breath focus helps you concentrate on slow deep breathing and let go of ideas and feelings that are distracting you. Also, it helps a lot if you tend to hold your stomach in.

As the first step you should find a quiet, nice place to sit or lie down. To begin, take a normal breath in. Next, take a deep breath: take slow, deep breaths in through your nose, and as you do this, let your chest and lower belly rise, allowing your stomach to fully stretch. Now, you can breathe out slowly through your nose or mouth.

After you've done the steps listed above, you can start taking controlled breaths every day. Sit comfortably with your eyes closed and take deep breaths. At the same time, think of helpful images and maybe a word or phrase that helps you relax.

You might want to try a few different ways to calm down and see which one works best for you. Pick a favorite spot where you can sit or lie down quietly and easily. Don’t try too hard, because that might make you tighten up, but don’t be too chilly either. To get the relaxation reaction, you need to shift your attention from things that are stressing you out to deeper, calmer rhythms. To make it feel more like a routine and form a habit, try to practice once or twice a day at the same time every time, for 10 to 20 minutes.[68]

The breathing technique to help with stress only takes a **few minutes** and you can do it anywhere to help with stress, anxiety, and fear. Adding it to your daily routine will help you the most. Being on your back in a chair, standing, or lying on a bed or yoga mat on the floor are all good ways to do it. If you can, take off any clothes that make it hard for you to breathe. If you are laying down, put your arms out to the sides, palms up, and stretch your legs straight or bend your knees so your feet are flat on the ground. If you're sitting down, put your arms on the chair arms and put both feet flat on the ground. Put your feet about hip-width apart no matter what situation you're in.

- Let your breath go as deep into your belly as it can go without pushing it.
- Take deep breaths in through your nose, and out through your mouth.
- Take slow, steady breaths in. It can help some people to count slowly from 1 to 5. At first, you might not be able to get to 5.
- Then, let it flow out slowly while you count from 1 to 5, if it helps
- Do this for at least 5 minutes[69]

---

[68] Harvard Health Publishing - https://www.health.harvard.edu/mind-and-mood/relaxation-techniques-breath-control-helps-quell-errant-stress-response (Published in July 2020)

[69] National Health Service - https://www.nhs.uk/mental-health/self-help/guides-tools-and-activities/breathing-exercises-for-stress (Reviewed in August 2022)

As time goes on, old air builds up, making it harder for the **diaphragm** to squeeze and bring in fresh air. Since the diaphragm isn't working as well as it should, the body starts to breathe with muscles in the neck, back, and chest. This means less oxygen in the blood and less energy for action and exercise. If you do breathe exercises regularly, they can help your lungs get rid of old air, raise your oxygen levels, and get your diaphragm back to its job of helping you breathe.

Pursed Lip breathing exercises that help you breathe make you breathe less frequently and keep your airways open longer. More air is able to flow in and out of your lungs so you can be more physically active. It's easy to do: just breathe in through your nose and then out through your mouth for at least twice as long, with your lips pursed.[70]

The importance of sleep[71]

Sleep is very **important** for your health and happiness all through your life. What goes on in your mind while you sleep affects how you feel when you wake up. Although you sleep, your body is still trying to keep your brain and your body healthy.

Heart disease, high blood pressure, obesity, and stroke may be more likely to happen to people who don't get enough sleep or wake up a lot at night. It can also change the way you think, act, learn, work, and get along with other people.

7 to 9 hours of sleep a night is what experts say people should get.

Adults who sleep less than 7 hours a night may have more health problems, while sleeping more than 9 hours a night is not always bad for you and can be helpful for sick people, young adults, and people who are recovering from not getting enough sleep.

---

[70] American Lung Association - https://www.lung.org/lung-health-diseases/wellness/breathing-exercises (Updated in November 2022)

[71] National Heart, Lung, and Blood Institute - https://www.nhlbi.nih.gov/health/sleep (Updated in March 2022)

There are **clocks** inside your body that tell you when to wake up and when to go to sleep. The rounds of these clocks are about 24 hours long. A lot of things, like light and darkness, affect these clocks, as well as sleep routines. Once you're asleep, you go through the stages of sleep in a regular way throughout the night.
Some people may have a different body clock than you do, that's why people wake up at different times and stay up late at different times. One example is that it is normal for many kids to want to go to bed and wake up later than adults.
If you follow a natural routine of days and nights, light signals from your eyes tell your brain that it's daytime. However, artificial light can mess up this process, so bright artificial light in the late evening can mess up this process and stop your brain from releasing melatonin, and this can make it harder to fall asleep. Bright artificial light comes from things like a TV screen, a smartphone, or an alarm clock that is very bright. Some people block some of the blue light from these gadgets with hardware or software.

Some **habits** that can help you **sleep better**[72]:

- Be consistent. Every night and every morning, even on the weekends, go to bed and wake up at a similar time
- Make sure your bedroom is at a good temperature, dark, quiet, and relaxing
- Keep electronics like TVs, computers, and cell phones out of the bedroom
- Don't eat or drink a lot of caffeine or alcohol before bed
- Get some exercise. Being busy during the day can make it easier for you to fall asleep at night

---

[72] Centers for Disease Control and Prevention - https://www.cdc.gov/sleep/about_sleep/sleep_hygiene.html (Reviewed in September 2022)

Some people have issues with their sleep-wake cycle, which means that their brains don't keep them awake or asleep at the right time. They might have one of these sleep problems.
People with **insomnia** have trouble either getting to sleep or staying asleep. They might not get enough good sleep or not enough sleep at all because of this. When they wake up, they might not feel refreshed.
People with **narcolepsy** get very sleepy during the day. Muscle weakness may also be a sign of the condition.

Do you ever wonder if taking naps is good for you? A lot of studies show that taking naps helps people learn, do better and be less sleepy during the day. Naps can help shift workers be more alert and quicker to respond. It's been found that a 20-minute nap is best. When you take a short nap like this, your mind and body can rest without falling asleep deeply. You might not feel as sleepy when you wake up if you drink a small amount of caffeine before your nap. This is because caffeine takes some time to work on your body. If you can't take a nap, being outside in the sun can help you restore energy.[73]

Cold showers[74]

It might be a good thing if you run out of hot water in the shower. Even if it's only for a few minutes, a cold shower can help you heal, recover, and feel better in general. This is especially true after working out.
Cold therapy, also known as **cryotherapy**, cools the body's tissues with cold temperature for therapeutic reasons.
Cold showers are not the primary treatment for any conditions, and there isn't a lot of solid study on cold therapy yet. A quick blast of cold water, on the other hand, can help ease symptoms.

---

[73] National Sleep Foundation - https://www.thensf.org/the-benefits-of-napping (Published in May 2021)
[74] University of California - https://www.uclahealth.org/news/6-cold-shower-benefits-consider (Published in January 2023)

Taking cold showers may:

- Keep from getting **colds**: taking a hot shower and then a cold shower, even for a short time, might protect you from viruses that are going around. The shock of cold water can wake up leukocytes, which are blood cells that fight off illness. A Dutch study found that people who took cold showers for 30, 60, or 90 seconds every day for 90 days missed work 29% less often than people who didn't take cold showers.
- Help with **depression** symptoms: Not much study has been done on how cold water therapy affects depression, but the studies that have been done so far show some good results. In one clinical study, people who took cold showers every day for a few months said they felt less depressed. More study shows that cold water may make you feel better and less anxious.
- Better **blood flow**: being in cold water makes your body work harder to keep its core temperature steady, putting it into "survival mode". This makes your body send more blood to the muscles.
- Speed up your **metabolism**: when you take a cold shower, your body uses energy to stay warm. It's possible that a few calories will be burned and your metabolism will speed up. But don't give up on your plan to eat well and exercise right away—there isn't much study on this benefit yet.
- Lower **inflammation** and stop muscle soreness: cold therapy makes your blood vessels narrow, which is called vasoconstriction, and when that happens, blood flows to the core and most important parts of your body. During the process, the blood automatically gets more oxygen and nutrients. Vasodilation means that the blood vessels get bigger, which brings fresh blood back to the tissues. As it moves back, it helps get rid of inflammation and soreness.
- Remove localized **pain**: cold treatment reduces inflammation, which takes away pain, but it also changes how your brain perceives pain by slowing down nerve signals that go to your brain.

No research has been done on how often someone should take a cold shower. It's suggested that you use cold treatment after working out. For example, if you work out every day, you can take a cold shower every day.

Here are some **tips** for taking cold showers:

- Don't let the water get above 60 degrees Fahrenheit (15 degrees Celsius): When you take a shower at home, make it as cold as you can
- Go slowly. Begin with 30 seconds of cold water. Work up to 1 minute until you can take a 2- to 3-minute cold shower
- Switch between hot and cold: It includes taking a 3-minute hot shower and then a 1-minute cold shower. Do it 3 times, and each time end with the cold

For most healthy people, taking a cold shower is **safe** and won't hurt them, but if you're worried, talk to your doctor.

Ways to become smarter[75]

Pumping iron can make your muscles bigger, and physical training can make you more durable. Can you change or get better by working out your brain? This isn't a silly question, since most people lose their mental abilities as they get older.

However, it turns out that some of the things you do every day can actually make you smarter.

- Your brain will work better if you **work out** often. The brain gets more blood when you exercise, which is like bringing food to the brain. This changes the brain at every level, from the chemical level to the behavioral level. Neurogenesis, the process by which new brain cells, or neurons, are made, is enhanced by exercise. Your brain's plasticity also gets better when you work out.

---

[75] Business Insider - https://www.insider.com/how-to-become-smarter-2018-7 (Published in July 2018)

- If you want to keep your brain active, **try dancing or golf**. Pick something that makes your brain and body work together. Because you have to think and move while doing things like dancing and golf, they can be very good for your brain. A study from 2003 in the New England Journal of Medicine showed that dancing and some other activities might help lower the risk of getting dementia.
- You might get smarter if you **learn in the same way that smart people do**. It may seem obvious, but learning how smart people think and learn can help you use the same methods to get smarter.
- You might get smarter if you **hang out with smart people**. The kids who had a smarter best friend in middle school were also smarter themselves by the time they got to high school. Having a smart partner can make you smarter because they introduce you to new things, ideas, and often smart new people.
- Paying attention to **one thing at a time** will help your brain work better. As much as you might think that doing a lot of things at once will help you get more done, it won't. A former psychology professor at Stanford University said that people who do multiple things at once have trouble with many cognitive tasks because they can't separate what's important from what's not. Try to get your mind back on the task of focusing on one thing at a time.
- You might get smarter if you **learn a new language**. People probably don't find it that strange that learning more than one language can be great for your brain. Using both languages regularly can help build up the part of your brain that helps you switch between languages and focus on the one you're speaking. There is also a study that showed people with Alzheimer's who spoke two languages seemed to handle the disease better than people who spoke only one language. They worked at about the same level, even though the brains of the bilingual patients had more damage.

In the end, you still can't be smarter than your natural brain. Put on your shorts and go work out instead of taking smart drugs and vitamins. Brain training might be a good idea for people over 60 and do everything with your friends.

Diseases

"Diseases are the tax on pleasures"
John Ray (Naturalist, 1700)

As for Cambridge Dictionary, a disease is an illness of people, animals, plants, etc., caused by infection or a failure of health rather than by an accident.
The origin of the word comes from Middle English, in the sense '**lack of ease**; inconvenience'.

Infectious diseases[76]

It is possible for pathogens, which are dangerous organisms that get into your body from the outside, to cause infectious diseases. Infectious diseases are caused by pathogens like viruses, bacteria, fungi, and parasites, and very rarely prions. You can get diseases from other people, bug bites, food, drink, or soil that has been tainted.

---

[76] Cleveland Clinic - https://my.clevelandclinic.org/health/diseases/17724-infectious-diseases (Reviewed in June 2022)

Viral infections. Viruses are made up of DNA or RNA that is wrapped in a protected shell. They are much smaller than your cells and can't reproduce on their own. They get into your cells and use the machinery inside them to make more copies of themselves.

- Cold: You have to let a cold run its course because there is no fix. In 7 to 10 days, most colds go away on their own and don't become something worse. As a common cold treatment, medicines can help ease your symptoms and keep you relaxed until you get better.
- The flu (influenza): Some flu symptoms, like a stuffy nose and cough, are similar to those of the common cold. However, cold symptoms are generally mild, while flu symptoms can be very bad and cause serious problems. In the Northern Hemisphere, flu season lasts from October to May, and between December and February is usually when the most cases happen, or "peak".
  How do I deal with flu symptoms? Rest, drinking water or broth to stay hydrated, and using heat packs or hot water bottles can help with aching muscles.
  Getting the flu shot every year is the best way to stay healthy and avoid getting the flu. You need to get a flu shot every year because the flu virus can change a little bit each year. Getting a flu shot lowers your risk of getting really sick, even if you get sick with a different strain of flu than the one in the vaccine.
- COVID-19: You can only be sure if you have the flu or COVID-19 by getting tested. This is because their symptoms are very identical.
- Stomach flu (gastroenteritis): The main sign of gastroenteritis is diarrhea, which can make you lose water. To feel better faster, rest and drink lots of water are the most important things you can do.

Bacterial infections. Bacteria have only one cell, and their DNA code provides their instructions. There are bacteria all around us, on our skin and inside our bodies. There are trillions of bacteria living in our bodies, and many of them are safe or even helpful. They help keep inflammation and disease in check, but some others give off toxins that can make you sick.

The best care is to use antibiotic medicines wisely. To make sure you get the best treatment when you're sick, protect yourself from harm caused by using antibiotics too often, and fight drug resistance. Antibiotics DO NOT kill viruses, so only take them if you need to. If you do need to take antibiotics, follow the directions exactly and finish the full course even if your symptoms go away.

- Salmonella: the most common type of food poisoning in the U.S, and it gives you gastroenteritis. Salmonella is much less likely to happen if you follow safe ways to prepare food and are careful around animals. Salmonella bacteria in food are killed by cooking and processing.
- Tuberculosis: Tuberculosis is a viral disease that can make your lungs or other tissues sick. It usually affects your lungs, but it can happen to other parts of your body too. Most of the time, you need to be around someone who has active TB for a long time before you get it yourself.
- Sexually Transmitted Infections (STIs): These are diseases or infections that you can get from any kind of sexual contact with your mouth, anus, vagina, or penis. Itching and burning around your private area are common signs of a STI. You can lower this chance by using a latex condom, being careful about who you sleep with, and getting checked for STIs often.
- Escherichia coli (E. coli): As long as a person is healthy, this bacterium should be present in their gut. This bacterium is usually not dangerous. It helps your body break down food, but some types of E. coli can make you sick with diarrhea, stomach cramps, pain, and a low-grade fever. Some E. coli infections can be dangerous. Washing your hands frequently is the most important care you can take to avoid getting E. coli.

Fungal infections. Fungi, similarly to bacteria, come in many forms. They are on your body and inside it. You can get sick if your fungi get too big or if dangerous fungi get into your body through your mouth, nose, or a cut on your skin.

- Ringworm (like athlete's foot): You might be shocked to learn that ringworm is caused by a fungus, not a worm. Fungi like places that are warm and damp, like locker rooms and public showers. Your skin would get the red, itchy, ring-shaped skin plaque (a type of bumpy rash) that these infections are known for. To avoid getting ringworm, make sure you change your socks and underwear every day or more often if they get dirty or wet, take a shower right after contact sports, wear sandals to the pool and in public locker rooms and showers, dry your skin well after showering, especially between your toes, and don't share towels.
- Vaginal candidiasis (vaginal yeast infection): As a fungus, yeast is one kind, and candida is one kind of yeast. If you have a yeast infection, the outside of your vagina (vulva) will burn, itch, and turn red. Your vaginal discharge will also change. Most of the time, you can avoid getting vaginal yeast infections by not washing the inside of your vagina (this can kill the bacteria that control fungus), not using feminine deodorants, not using scented tampons or pads, taking off your wet clothes, and using sexual lubricants that are water-based.

Parasitic infections. Parasites live and reproduce inside the bodies of other living things. Worms and some single-celled organisms (protozoa) are examples of parasites.

A lot of infectious diseases go away on their own, but some can make you sick for a long time.
When it comes to viral diseases, there are a lot of different **ways they can spread**, but luckily, there are easy ways to avoid getting infections most of the time.

It's easy for germs to get into your body through your mouth, nose, and cuts.
Diseases can spread:

- When you cough or sneeze from one person to another. Some coughing or sneezing droplets can stay in the air for a long time
- Kissing, oral, anal, or vaginal sex
- Sharing tools or cups with other people
- When you touch poop from a person or animal
- On things like doorknobs, phones, and counters
- When you get bitten by a bug or an animal
- When you eat or drink something that is contaminated or not properly prepared
- When you work with contaminated soil or sand, like when you garden

Sexually transmitted diseases

In US in 2019, the top 5 new cases of infectious diseases per 100,000 population are:[77]

- Chlamydia: 553
- Gonorrhea: 188
- Syphilis: 40
- Salmonella: 18
- Lyme disease: 11

It's quite relevant to highlight that the first 3, which are the dominant, are sexually transmitted diseases.
Sexual interaction, such as oral, vaginal, and anal sex, is known to spread **more than 30 types** of bacteria, viruses, and parasites. These are known as sexually transmitted diseases (STIs). There are 8 bacteria that are most often linked to STIs, and only 4 of them can be cured right now: syphilis, gonorrhea, chlamydia, and trichomoniasis. The other 4 viruses

---

[77] Centers for Disease Control and Prevention - https://www.cdc.gov/nchs/data/hus/2020-2021/IDNotif.pdf (Reviewed in September 2023)

that can't be cured are hepatitis B, HIV, the human papillomavirus (HPV), and herpes simplex virus (HSV).

Every day, more than **1 million STIs are spread**. In 2016, it was estimated that more than 490 million people had genital herpes, about 300 million women had an HPV infection, and about 296 million people around the world have chronic hepatitis B.

Sexually transmitted infections (STIs) can have bad effects that **last longer** than the illness itself.
STIs like syphilis, herpes, and gonorrhea can make getting HIV more likely. STIs can be passed from mother to child, which can lead to stillbirth, newborn death, low birth weight, being born early, sepsis, neonatal conjunctivitis, and birth defects. HPV infections are the main reason men who have sex with other men get cervical and anal cancer. About 820,000 people died from hepatitis B in 2019, mostly from cirrhosis and hepatocellular cancer. STIs like gonorrhea and chlamydia are a big reason why women get pelvic inflammatory disease and can't have children.

STIs often don't cause any **symptoms**. Symptoms can be vague when they show up, and at least one STI can live in three different body parts. This makes it hard to diagnose STIs, and people are often treated for two or more of them at the same time.

Condoms are one of the best ways to avoid getting STI as long as they are used properly and regularly. Condoms are very good at keeping you safe, but they don't protect against STIs that cause extra-genital ulcers, like syphilis and genital herpes. With all types of sex, condoms should be used whenever possible.
Two viral STIs, hepatitis B and HPV, have **vaccines** that are safe and very successful. These medicines are big steps forward in the fight against STIs. In 111 countries, mostly high- and middle-income ones, the HPV vaccine had become a standard part of immunization programs by the end of 2020. To get rid of cervical cancer as a global public health issue,

high coverage goals must be met by 2030 for HPV vaccination, screening for and treatment of precancerous lesions, and cancer management.

5 of the world's deadliest infectious diseases[78]

The World Health Organization (WHO) says that about 10 million people got **tuberculosis (TB)** in 2018, and about 1.5 million people died. It's still the most common cause of death from a single infectious agent, even though it can be cured and stopped, and it's one of the top 10 reasons people die around the world.
Bacteria that cause TB are spread through coughs and sneezes. Antibiotics can help treat it, but multidrug-resistant and extensively drug-resistant TB can happen if the drugs aren't used correctly or are being handled. The WHO calls multidrug-resistant tuberculosis a public health disaster, and in 2016, it spread to nearly 500,000 people around the world. Treatment for these strains takes a long time and costs a lot of money.

The virus that causes **measles** is very contagious and very dangerous. It is spread through coughs, sneezes, and close touch. It can live in the air for two hours and is so contagious that up to 90% of people who are close to someone who has it will get it if they are not already protected. Many children around the world get a safe and effective vaccine before they turn 1 year old, resulting in 2018 86% of children to get this vaccine.
But it still kills a lot of people in poor countries, mostly in Africa and Asia, reaching 140,000 deaths globally in 2018. More than 95% of these deaths happen in places where people don't make much money and the health system isn't very good.

Malaria can be controlled, as history has shown. It was prevalent in Western Europe and the US but wiped out by the mid-1930s and 1951 respectively. However, there were still an estimated 228 million cases

[78] World Economic Forum - https://www.weforum.org/agenda/2020/04/covid-19-infectious-diseases-tuberculosis-measles-malaria (Published in April 2020)

and 405,000 deaths around the world in 2018. Most of these (94%) happened in the Africa region, with children under 5 being the most at risk.

The Bill & Melinda Gates Foundation says that since 2000, the number of malaria deaths has dropped by half, but the Anopheline mosquito type is becoming less sensitive to insecticides, and the parasite it spreads is also becoming less sensitive to certain drugs. Vector control, like insecticide-treated nets and indoor residual sprays, is an important first line of defense. But as the rate of death reduction slows, it's time to find new and creative ways to get rid of the disease, like using epidemiological data for planning and analysis.

Every year, around winter time, a lot of people get the **flu**. A few bad days in bed are what most people get out of it. However, people in high-risk groups, like pregnant women, the elderly, and people who have long-term health problems, can die from it.

The WHO says that between 3 and 5 million people get serious flu every year, and up to 650,000 die. This can put a huge load on healthcare systems during times of high infection (health workers are more likely to get the disease), and it also has an impact on the economy as schools and workplaces deal with missing students and staff.

Cholera and **dysentery** may sound like diseases that killed a lot of people in the 1800s, but the reality is actually very different. It's the second most common cause of death in young children, after acute respiratory illnesses. Every year, diarrhea kills about 525,000 children under 5 years old.

It's usually caused by an illness of the intestines, which can be bacterial, viral, or parasitic. It's often spread from person to person through bad hygiene or contaminated food or water, which is worst in the world's poorest areas. The WHO says that around the world, 780 million people do not have access to clean water for drinking and 2.5 billion do not have good hygiene.

COVID-19 pandemic

The COVID-19, which is caused by SARS-CoV-2 virus, first showed up in late 2019 and quickly spread around the world.

As of January 2020, the World Health Organization (WHO) said that the COVID-19 spread was a public health emergency of international concern (PHEIC). Then, the COVID-19 spread was called a **pandemic** by the Director-General of WHO in March 2020. Vaccines that were given all over the world starting in 2021 have greatly lessened the spread of COVID-19 since then, even though new strains that are easier to spread have appeared.

As of May 2023, the Director-General of WHO said that COVID-19 is no longer a PHEIC. He said that even though the population immunity level is better and there are fewer hospitalizations and deaths, it is still unclear how the SARS-CoV-2 virus will change.

As of June 2023, SARS-CoV-2 is still going around, though not as strongly as before. In 2022, there have been waves of infections about every 2 to 3 months, with trends toward lower peak numbers of cases, hospitalizations, ICU admissions, and deaths.[79]

Globally, as of November 2023, there have been 772 million confirmed cases of COVID-19, including 7 million deaths[80]

---

[79] European Centre for Disease Prevention and Control - https://www.ecdc.europa.eu/en/covid-19/questions-answers/questions-answers-eu-situation (Updated in June 2023)

[80] World Health Organization - https://covid19.who.int (Accessed in May 2024)

For an updated status, or to check the current situations and trends worldwide or in specific countries, you can visit the WHO website: https://covid19.who.int

When a sick person sneezes, coughs, talks, or breathes close to other people, respiratory droplets and aerosols are the main ways that the **virus gets around**. People can breathe in droplets or get them in their mouths, noses, or eyes.
Getting a COVID-19 vaccine, washing, or sanitizing your hands often, and opening windows often to let more air in can all lower your risk of getting SARS-CoV-2.
Sometimes people with COVID-19 don't have any symptoms at all, while other people have fever, cough, sore throat, overall weakness, fatigue, muscle pain, and loss of smell and taste.
In the worst cases, pneumonia and acute respiratory distress syndrome can make it hard to breathe, and other problems can happen that could even be fatal.

People who have been infected with the COVID-19 virus may have long-term effects from their illness. These effects are called **Long COVID** or Post-COVID Conditions (PCC). Long COVID includes a wide range of signs, symptoms, and conditions that happen or get worse after an initial COVID-19 infection. Long COVID can mean a lot of different long-term health problems that can last for weeks, months, or even years.

Long COVID can develop to anyone who gets COVID, and a lot of work is being done to figure out why some people get Long COVID and others don't.

Study after study has shown that the following groups of people may be more likely to get Long COVID:

- People who get severely ill from COVID, especially those who need hospital care
- People who have underlying health conditions
- People who aren't vaccinated against COVID
- People who experience multisystem inflammatory syndrome (MIS) during or after COVID illness
- People who have COVID more than once[81]

How to boost your immune system[82]

It sounds good to be able to boost your immune system, but for a number of reasons, it has been hard to do so. That's right, the defense system is a system, not a single thing. Balance and unity are needed for it to work well. Researchers still don't know a lot about how the immune system works and how **all of its parts work together**. At this point, there are no scientifically proven straight links between how you live your life and having a stronger immune system.

What that does not mean, though, is that the effects of lifestyle on the immune system are not interesting and should not be researched. Diet, exercise, age, psychological stress, and other things are being studied to see how they affect the immune system in both animals and people.

---

[81] U.S. Department of Health and Human Services (HHS) - https://wecandothis.hhs.gov/resource/facts-about-covid-19-and-the-vaccines (Reviewed in June 2023)

[82] Harvard Health Publishing - https://www.health.harvard.edu/staying-healthy/how-to-boost-your-immune-system (Published in March 2024)

For now, it makes sense to follow general healthy-living tips because they are likely to boost the immune system and have other health benefits that have been shown to work, such as:

- **Don't smoke.**
- Eat a diet high in **fruits** and **vegetables**: There is some proof that not getting enough of some micronutrients, like zinc, selenium, iron, copper, folic acid, vitamins A, B6, C, and E, can change how the immune system works. So, if you think that your food isn't giving you all the micronutrients you need—maybe because you don't like vegetables—taking a daily multivitamin and mineral supplement may help your health in more ways than one. Taking huge amounts of a single vitamin doesn't help. It's not always better to have more.
- **Exercise** regularly.
- Maintain a healthy **weight.**
- If you drink **alcohol**, drink only in moderation.
- Get adequate **sleep.**
- Take steps to **avoid infection**, like washing your hands a lot and cooking meat all the way through. Following the traditional way of cooking and eating raw meat is the best advice. Make sure the raw meat is very fresh and only buy it from a trustworthy butcher who knows this is how it will be eaten. Also, it's important to keep raw meat away from ready-to-eat foods that won't be cooked because this makes it less likely that cross-contamination will happen, which can happen.
- Try to minimize **stress**: Mind and body are closely connected, and modern science has come to understand this. Emotional worry can cause a lot of different health problems, from stomach problems and hives to heart disease. Even though it's hard, experts are working hard to figure out how stress affects immune function.
- Keep current with all recommended **vaccines**. A vaccine makes your immune system ready to fight off germs before they get into your body.

It's easy to find **pills and plant remedies** in stores that say they "support immunity" or improve the health of your immune system in some other way. Even though some preparations have been shown to change some parts of how the immune system works, there is still no proof that they actually make you less likely to get sick or get an illness. It is still very hard to prove whether a plant or any other substance can boost immunity.

Suggested vaccination[83]

A simple, safe, and effective way to protect yourself from dangerous diseases before you get them is to get a vaccine. It boosts your immune system and uses your body's natural defenses to make you less likely to get certain infections.

Getting a vaccine makes your immune system **produce antibodies**, just like it does when you get a sickness. A vaccine, on the other hand, only has viruses or bacteria that have been killed or weakened. This means that it does not cause the disease or put you at risk for its effects.

Getting a vaccine is the best way to keep people from getting sick, and it's also one of the least expensive ways to improve public health. Most people have been vaccinated against many illnesses, and this has almost wiped out smallpox, polio, and many others.

These are the **regular shots** that everyone should make sure they have: **Tetanus, Diphtheria,** and **whooping cough** (also known as **pertussis**).

Adults who have never had a shot should get one, and after that, they should get either a Td (tetanus and diphtheria) or Tdap (tetanus, diphtheria, and pertussis) shot every 10 years.

There are vaccines for 18 diseases that are very dangerous or can kill you, so you may need other vaccines too, depending on your age, job, trip plans, and health.

---

[83] Centers for Disease Control and Prevention - https://www.cdc.gov/vaccines/adults/rec-vac/index.html (Reviewed in September 2023)

Any vaccine can have side effects, but most of the time they are mild (like a sore arm or a low-grade fever) and go away in a few days.

Can being too clean weaken your immune system?[84]

There is **no scientific proof** that being very clean is bad for your immune system.
People probably got the idea that washing your hands a lot weakens your immune system from something called the **hygiene hypothesis**. This hypothesis states that being around more viruses, germs, and other pathogens when they are young makes the immune systems stronger.
There is still disagreement about this theory and how important it is to keep yourself clean.

Studies have shown over and over that one of the best ways to stop the spread of dangerous diseases is to keep your **hands clean**.
The CDC says to wash your hands with soap and water after being in public or after blowing your nose, coughing, or sneezing to stop the spread of contagious diseases. If you need to wash your hands but soap and water aren't available, use a hand sanitizer made with at least 60% alcohol.
Your skin can get dried or cracked from washing and sanitizing your hands a lot, so you might want to use a good lotion after you wash your hands.
The CDC also says that you should clean areas in your home that you touch often, like doorknobs, light switches, countertops, and faucets.

---

[84] Cleveland Clinic - https://health.clevelandclinic.org/can-being-too-clean-weaken-your-immune-system (Published in May 2020)

Winter illness[85]

Respiratory viruses tend to spread a lot in the fall and winter.
But why does cold weather usually mean flu and cold season? Experts often say that changes in human behavior are to blame. For example, when it's cold outside, people **stay inside**, which makes it easier for germs to spread.

Moreover, a new study in The Journal of Allergy and Clinical Immunology shows that our **noses** may hold the key to another explanation. The nose is the body's main connection to the outside world, so it has defenses against viruses and germs that stop them in their tracks. They found that when the nose finds bacteria, it sends out a lot of tiny fluid-filled sacs that are supposed to attack and kill the bacteria.
For the study, researchers set the healthy volunteers' nasal temperatures at about 74°F (23°C), and others at about 40°F (4°C). In the colder situation, they found that the temperature inside the nose dropped by about 9°F (-13°C). Next, they put nasal cell samples through a similar drop in temperature in the lab to see what would happen in the nose in a cold environment. At the lower temperature, they found that the immune reaction was slowed down a lot.
In other words, this natural immune defense system will work better if you can keep the air inside your nose warmer. There may be yet another reason to wear masks.
Researchers might be able to stop more viral illnesses before they start if they can find a way to boost the nose's natural immune response, even when it's cold outside.

---

[85] Time - https://time.com/6238816/why-viruses-spread-in-cold-weather (Published in December 2022)

Does air conditioning make you ill?[86]

The Spanish Pneumology Society says that summer is when 20% of colds happen and when half of sick days are taken because of colds.
If you keep your Air Conditioner (AC) in good shape, it won't make you sick. **Sick building syndrome**, on the other hand, can be caused by pathogens, poor ventilation, dust, fabric fibers in the air, fumes, or a unit that hasn't been kept well.
In their most basic form, air fans cool the air by pulling in hot air from that room. Once the air is cool, fans inside the unit push it out into the room.

The room's dust particles **may cause** allergic reactions like stuffy or runny noses, itchy eyes, and rashes as they move around and get spread. Also, germs that are in the air, like the SARS-CoV-2 virus, have a higher chance of being breathed in because they are always moving. Some of these problems may make lung diseases like asthma worse. Some AC units with a HEPA (High Efficiency Particulate Air) screen can lower this risk.
Additionally, if the unit isn't regularly kept, mold spores can grow and spread throughout the room, which can make you feel sick and cause breathing problems, especially if you are allergic to or sensitive to mold. People who don't take care of their air conditioners can get legionnaires' disease, a type of pneumonia that can be very dangerous, in which the air sacs fill with pus caused by bacteria. Usually, symptoms show up between 2 and 14 days.

If you stay in a room with air conditioning for a long time, these are some of the most common **signs** of sick building syndrome: getting headaches, having a runny nose, having dry, itchy skin, having dry, sore eyes or throat, coughing or wheezing, rashes, being tired, and having trouble focusing.

---

[86] MyHSN - https://www.myhsn.co.uk/whats-hot/does-air-conditioning-really-give-you-a-cold (Accessed in May 2024)

If these things are happening to you, **you should**:

- Open windows to let more air in.
- Set a temperature and don't change it often during the day.
- Take breaks from your computer screen often.
- Go outside for extra fresh air during lunch and other breaks.
- Don't turn the air conditioner down below 77°F (25°C). Your comfort won't get better, but the amount of energy you use (which will raise also the energy cost) and the damage to your health will go through the roof. When the temperature difference between the dry area (below 30% relative humidity) and the street temperature is more than 50°F (10°C), problems start to happen. In the summer, 79°F (26°C) is usually the best setting to aim for.[87]
- Use a humidifier.

Fever[88]

A fever is when your body temperature is too high, and it generally means that something is going wrong in the body. Getting exercise, being outside in the heat, and getting common vaccines can all raise body temperature.

A fever by itself does not mean you are sick. Instead, it's a sign that something is wrong with the body.

A fever is usually defined to be **100.4°F (38°C)** or higher.

Paracetamol is a popular drug that can help with pain and fevers caused by colds and flu, and it's generally mixed with other molecules, like cold and flu remedies or some painkillers. After 1 hour, paracetamol should

[87] Endesa - https://www.endesa.com/en/blogs/endesa-s-blog/air-conditioning/what-happens-if-you-turn-the-air-conditioning-down-too-low (Published in July 2019)

[88] John Hopkins Medicine - https://www.hopkinsmedicine.org/health/conditions-and-diseases/fever (Accessed in May 2024)

start to work, and the effects generally last for several hours. If the amount recommended doesn't help your symptoms, don't take more.

Fight inflammation[89]

People who have sprained their ankle, cut themselves while cutting veggies, or been stung by a bee can see what inflammation is like. That it hurts, turns red, swells, and gets hot is the body's way of protecting itself against germs like bacteria and fixing damaged tissue. Inflammation from an infection like a cold, the flu, or COVID-19 is less visible, but it works in the same way.

Acute inflammation is the body's quick response system that gets rid of harmful invaders and restores balance, and it happens when the body is hurt or infected. A burst of chemicals that sound the alarm brings a huge number of white blood cells to the wound. There are cells that fight off the invaders and cells that fix the damage caused by the war. Acute soreness usually goes away quickly, in a few hours to a few days.
Acute inflammation has clear and instant signs like redness, pain, warmth, and swelling.

In the same way, **chronic inflammation** can start when the body tries to get rid of things that its immune system sees as alien invaders, but this inflammation can last for a long time, even if the threat isn't really dangerous to your health. When someone has an autoimmune disease, such as rheumatoid arthritis, lupus, type 1 diabetes, ulcerative colitis, or multiple sclerosis, their body attacks their own tissues as if they were foreign, which causes inflammation that hurts them.
This low-grade inflammation may stay under the surface for a long time, and it can be caused by bad habits like smoking, eating poorly, drinking alcohol, being inactive, stress, and gaining weight.
Chronic inflammation happens more slowly and in a more subtle way. When symptoms do show up, they may include tiredness, aches and

---

[89] Harvard Health Publishing - https://www.health.harvard.edu/staying-healthy/all-about-inflammation (Published in June 2020)

pains in the muscles and joints, weight gain, headaches, and skin rashes. Other symptoms may include constipation, diarrhea, and other problems with the digestive system.

All of the following **diseases can be contributed** by inflammation and the harmful chemicals it makes: cancer, Alzheimer's and other types of dementia, high blood pressure, heart disease, stroke, type 2 diabetes, allergies and asthma, skin problems like acne, eczema, and psoriasis, and arthritis.

Here are some ways to **fight inflammation** and all of its bad effects on the body:

- To reduce inflammation, eat a lot of fruits, veggies, nuts, whole grains, healthy oils, and fatty fish like salmon, sardines, and tuna. Cut back on sugary and starchy foods like soda and candy, as well as processed carbs like cookies and pie. A lot of these principles are part of the Mediterranean diet.
- Each week, try to do at least 150 minutes of aerobic exercise and at least 2 muscle strength training.
- Watch your weight by eating right and working out.
- Get at least 7 to 9 hours of sleep every night.
- Give up smoking and drink no more than 1 or 2 drinks a day.
- Deep breathing, meditation, and yoga are all relaxing exercises that can help you deal with long-term stress.

Autoimmune diseases[90-91]

When the immune system is strong, it protects the body from getting sick, but when the **immune system doesn't work right**, it affects healthy cells, tissues, and organs. These attacks can happen in any part of the body and are known as autoimmune diseases. They can make it harder for the body to work and can even be life-threatening.

There are **more than 80 autoimmune illnesses** that scientists know about. Some are well known, like type 1 diabetes, multiple sclerosis, lupus, and rheumatoid arthritis. Others are not as common and can be hard to identify. People with rare inflammatory diseases may suffer for years before they get a correct diagnosis, and most of these illnesses can't be cured, so they need to be treated for the rest of their life just to ease the effects.

More people are getting autoimmune diseases, but **no one knows why**, since the causes of these diseases are also still a secret and studies show that these diseases are probably caused by genetic and environmental factors interacting with each other.

They are more likely to happen with the following factors:

- There is no doubt that **genes** play a part in autoimmune disease, but scientists still don't fully understand how.
- **Women** are more likely to get autoimmune diseases, but doctors don't know why either. One idea is that women may be because their hormone levels are higher, especially when they are trying to have a baby.
- What role do **infections** and diseases play? It's thought by many experts that this is what causes rheumatoid arthritis, an autoimmune disease that hurts the joints. Also, people who

[90] John Hopkins Medicine - https://www.hopkinsmedicine.org/health/wellness-and-prevention/autoimmune-disease-why-is-my-immune-system-attacking-itself (Accessed in May 2024)

[91] National Institute of Environmental Health Sciences - https://www.niehs.nih.gov/health/topics/conditions/autoimmune/index.cfm (Accessed in May 2024)

have had strep throat often go on to get psoriasis, an autoimmune disease that makes patches of thick, scaly skin appear.

- Certain **races** and ethnicities
- Scientists believe that **damage** may play a part in some types of autoimmune diseases, like psoriatic arthritis, which affects the joints of some people with psoriasis. Researchers have found that when tendons, which connect muscle to bone, get damaged in parts of the body that are under a lot of stress, an autoimmune response takes place.

Diabetes mellitus[92]

Diabetes mellitus is the full name of this known disease, generally just called "diabetes”. The name diabetes mellitus comes from the Greek word diabetes, which means "to pass through," and the Latin word mellitus, which means "honeyed" or "sweet”. This is because people with diabetes have **too much sugar** in their blood and urine. Literature from the time of the Greeks, Chinese, Egyptians, Indians, and Persians shows that these people had noticed this sweet taste in pee. Apollonius of Memphis most likely came up with the word "diabetes" around 250 BC. Afterwards, it was also called the "pissing evil" in the 1600s.

Diabetes is a chronic disease that changes how your body turns food into energy.

A lot of the food you eat is turned by your body into **glucose**, which is a type of sugar, and then stored in your blood. Then pancreas makes **insulin** when your blood sugar levels rise, and insulin is like a key that lets the sugar from your blood into your cells so they can be used as energy.

If you have diabetes, your body either doesn't make enough insulin or can't use it properly. If your cells stop reacting to insulin or there isn't

[92] Centers for Disease Control and Prevention - https://www.cdc.gov/diabetes/basics/diabetes.html (Reviewed in September 2023)

enough of it, too much sugar stays in your blood. Some of the bad health effects that can happen over time are heart disease, eye loss, and kidney disease.

Type 1 and Type 2 diabetes are the two main types. About 90% of people with diabetes have type 2. It takes years to develop and is most often found in adults, but kids, teens, and young adults are getting it too more and more. You might not have any signs, so you should get your blood sugar checked.

Making good changes to your **lifestyle**, like losing weight, eating well, and being active, can help you avoid or put off getting type 2 diabetes. In case you get it, there isn't a cure yet, but these lifestyle changes may still help in managing the disease.

Most people have **prediabetes** before they get type 2 diabetes, which means that their blood sugar is higher than usual but not yet high enough to be diagnosed with diabetes. More than 80% of adults in the US who have prediabetes don't know they have it. That's 96 million people. Prediabetes can be fixed, which is good news.
Don't believe too much the "pre" part because prediabetes is a very bad health problem.
You might not know you have prediabetes for years. In other words, you probably won't know you have prediabetes until you start having major health issues. If you are overweight, 45 years or older, have a parent, brother, or sister with type 2 diabetes, are physically inactive less than 3 times a week, or have ever had gestational diabetes (diabetes during pregnancy) or given birth to a baby that weighed more than 9 pounds (4 kilograms), you should talk to your doctor about getting your blood sugar checked.
Ethnicity and race are also important. People of color, Hispanic or Latino Americans, American Indians, Pacific Islanders, and some Asian Americans are more likely to get it.

Are you ready to find out what your risk is? Check your chance of prediabetes in just 1 minute with this test made by the Centers for Disease Control and Prevention:
https://www.cdc.gov/prediabetes/risktest/index.html

Prediabetes is like a road split: type 2 diabetes is more likely to happen if you don't do anything about it. In conclusion, Prediabetes = **PreventDiabetes** [93]

Allergies[94]

Around the world, allergies are one of the **most common chronic illnesses**. Having allergy symptoms can make you unhappy or even put you at risk for reactions that could kill you.
The top allergy doctors say that an allergic reaction starts in the immune system. When you have an allergy, your immune system thinks that a substance that is normally safe is an invader, so the Immunoglobulin E (IgE) antibodies respond too strongly to the allergen. When these antibodies go to cells, they make histamine and other chemicals that cause an allergic response.

---

[93] Centers for Disease Control and Prevention - https://www.cdc.gov/diabetes/library/features/truth-about-prediabetes.html (Reviewed in July 2022)

[94] American Academy of Allergy, Asthma, and Immunology - https://www.aaaai.org/Conditions-Treatments/Allergies/Allergies-Overview (Accessed in May 2024)

Allergic responses are caused by a number of different **allergens**. pollen, dust mites, food, insect stings, animal hair, mold, medicines, and latex are some of the most frequent.

People who are allergic often have **symptoms** in their nose, lungs, mouth, sinuses, ears, stomach lining, or skin. For some people, allergens can trigger asthma and in the worst situations, a response called anaphylaxis can happen, which can be life-threatening.
If someone has **anaphylaxis**, they need to see a doctor right away and get an adrenaline (epinephrine) shot, then they should also go to the emergency room of a hospital. It is possible to die from anaphylaxis if it is not handled properly.

It's hard to say what causes allergies to appear because it depends on your genes and the allergens you are exposed to and when.
But doctors say that in general, things that mess up your immune system, like puberty, pregnancy, short-term or long-term illnesses, or organ transplants, can make you more or less allergic to things you used to be okay with.
Luckily, there are some things that can be done to **delay** or even **stop** allergies or asthma from happening.
Between 4 and 6 months, babies can start eating things with only one ingredient, and this way of introducing food can be done every 3 to 5 days, depending on how ready the baby is for it at that time. This slow process gives parents or other caregiver time to find any food that causes an allergic reaction and get rid of it. After less allergenic foods have been accepted for 4 to 6 months, egg, dairy, peanut, tree nut, fish, and shellfish can be slowly added. In fact, waiting to give your baby these foods may make it more likely for them to develop allergies.
Because some substances in the air can cause allergy or asthma symptoms, limiting exposure to these substances early in life may delay or stop allergy or asthma symptoms. The best research for this is done on dust mites. Cover pillows and beds with zippered, "allergen-impermeable" covers, and wash your bedding once a week in hot water. The humidity inside should stay below 50%. If you can, you should get

rid of any rugs or upholstered furniture in your baby's room. The relationship between early life exposure to animals and the development of allergies and asthma is somewhat confusing and there are many factors to consider.[95]

People often "lose" their allergies or become "desensitized" to an allergen, especially around or after middle age, when their immune systems "quiet down," getting weaker and less active.[96]

Staying away from things that cause your allergies is the best way to deal with the symptoms.

Food intolerances[97]

Food intolerance is different to a food allergy, which causes symptoms such as itchy skin, wheezing or swelling of the lips, face, and eyes. Food intolerances can show up in many other ways, but the most common ones are diarrhea, bloating, farting, and stomach pain.

If you have food intolerance, you have **trouble digesting** certain foods or ingredients, so your body can’t break them down. It's not usually a big deal but eating something you're intolerant of can make you feel unwell.

If you have food intolerance instead of a food allergy, your immune system is not overreacting to certain types of food, which means you cannot have a serious allergic response.

The reason some people get food intolerances is unknown to experts.

---

[95] American Academy of Allergy, Asthma, and Immunology - https://www.aaaai.org/tools-for-the-public/conditions-library/allergies/prevention-of-allergies-and-asthma-in-children (Reviewed in January 2024)

[96] The New York Times - https://www.nytimes.com/2023/04/19/well/adult-allergies.html (Published in April 2023)

[97] National Health Service - https://www.nhs.uk/conditions/food-intolerance (Reviewed in November 2022)

If you're intolerant to certain foods, try to **avoid** or eat less of them, however you should not cut food out of your or your child's diet without first talking to a doctor or a nutritionist. This is because you or your child might not get enough of some minerals and vitamins that are very important for a child's body and growth.

Lactose intolerance is the most common type of food intolerance and this is when your body can't break down lactose, a sugar that is mostly found in milk and dairy products like yogurt and cheese. Some people can't break down lactose because their bodies don't make enough of the enzyme lactase.
People also often can't handle **gluten**, which is not the same as coeliac disease: people with celiac disease have immune systems that fight their own tissues when they eat gluten, and this hurts the small intestine, making it hard for the body to absorb nutrients properly. People who have non-celiac gluten intolerance have symptoms that are like those of celiac disease, but they don't test positive for celiac disease.

Fertility and children

"There is only one pretty child in the world, and every mother has it". — Chinese Proverb

The word pregnancy comes from Latin **praegnantem**, literally "before birth": prae- "before" + root of gnasci "be born".
An associated term for pregnancy is gravid, and "gravidus" comes from the Latin word meaning "heavy".

The thought of the baby that might come from a conception makes us all feel warm and fuzzy inside. So many people seem to have kids as part of their plan, and it's not hard to do, however conception is often called a "**miracle**" because it takes a lot of work for an egg to become fertilized.

Plain and simple, a woman must be about to ovulate at the same time that the sperm start their journey.
More than 100 million sperm are in a healthy man's ejaculation. Though it sounds like a lot, less than 40% are thought to be "normal" at the start of the trip, and millions will die, get lost, or swim in the wrong direction before they even get close to where the egg is waiting.
Once they get past the cervical mucus, the uterus, and the fallopian tubes, which are like minefields, only about 50 sperm make it to where the egg is. After that, they have to hope that this fussy egg is ready to go.
The egg can only be fertilized for 12 to 24 hours per cycle, but the few healthy sperm that are still alive can wait for the egg for up to 5 days.
Finally, if everything goes as planned, one lucky sperm will be able to reach the egg and fertilize it, and this will start a whole new set of problems.
Once the sperm gets into the ovum, the egg is fertilized and grows into a baby, but cells must divide and the baby must be implanted in order for conception to work. This is when the embryo attaches to the lining or wall of the uterus. It lasts for about 6 days after fertilization.
At this point, the embryo needs to stay alive, and the risk of miscarriage is largest right after it implants. Up to 50% of fertilized eggs may not make it, and many of these end in an "unnoticed miscarriage" that looks like a period.
It is thought that up to 20% of known pregnancies will end in miscarriage, and most of these will happen in the first three months.[98]

Once this works, it makes sense that there would be some **changes** in the woman body. After all, a pregnant body is full of hormones. Women who are pregnant make more estrogen in one day than women who are not pregnant do in a year.

---

[98] Planned Parenthood - https://www.plannedparenthood.org/learn/pregnancy/how-pregnancy-happens (Accessed in May 2024)

When a woman is pregnant, an extra organ called the placenta grows and makes hormones. The uterus of a woman is usually about the size of an orange, and it can get to be about the size of a watermelon by the third trimester, growing up to 500 times bigger.

Your heart gets bigger as well, to help pump all that extra blood around your body when you're pregnant. Your blood volume goes up by up to 50% to make sure the baby gets enough fresh blood.

The voice can also change. When levels of estrogen and progesterone rise, the vocal folds may swell. This can make it so that higher notes are lost and lower ones may come through.

A lot of women also say that their feet increase to a whole size bigger while they were having babies.

In the first trimester, pregnant women often have a stronger sense of smell, which can be a sign that they are actually pregnant. It could be a way for animals to help pregnant people stay away from foods that are bad for them. Hormonal changes during pregnancy may mess up a woman's sense of smell and taste, making her want strange foods. Cravings could also mean that both the mother and the baby are not getting enough of some nutrients. For example, wanting red meat could mean you don't have enough iron.

Stretch marks, which are usually lighter than regular skin, can show up on a pregnant body as it changes. Women can also get melasma, which makes the face look like it has dark spots all over it. The vagina can also change color. It's known as the Chadwick Sign when some women say their vagina turns purple or blue. Blue varicose veins also show up down there in about 10% of women, but they should go away a few weeks after giving birth.

Research shows that about 80% of women have memory problems, but it's not clear what could be making it happen. The late nights, being tired, and the stress of welcoming a new life into the world could be to blame.

Hearing a baby cry can make a pregnant woman start to breastfeed. It doesn't have to be her own baby, it all works automatically.

Pregnancy gingivitis is when a woman's hormones change in a way that makes her gums more likely to get plaque. This plaque can cause swelling, bleeding, and bad breath in the gums.
Because it can grow faster during pregnancy, hair may feel bigger and better, but women can also get hair on their back, face, belly, and other parts of their bodies.
Researchers found fetal cells in moms' brains a few years ago. It turns out that baby cells can move from the placenta into the mother's organs to help heal damaged tissues.
The pelvic bone splits apart during birth. Moreover, a thin band of cartilage and ligaments connects the pelvis to the lower body, and this band can sometimes come apart during childbirth.
It's possible for your partner to have some of the same symptoms, and this is known as couvade syndrome, or sensitive pregnancy. More study is needed to find out if it has psychological causes, but men have said that they had heartburn, abdominal pain, back pain, anxiety, and depression.
Most pregnancies last around 280 days, but the shortest and longest pregnancies that were still alive were 151 days and 375 days, respectively. A lot of women have longer births than you might think. While most women are only pregnant for 9 months, many say they were pregnant for 10 or 11 months.

From inside the womb, **babies** can hear their mom's words. Babies can hear sounds when they are about 18 weeks old. By 25 to 26 weeks, it can hear sounds better and react in the womb.
Also, babies can taste some foods while they are still there, so strong tastes like garlic can get through to them. In fact, babies are more likely to like carrot juice if their moms drank a lot of it while they were pregnant.
Babies can cry while they are still in the womb, and this was found by chance when researchers looked at pregnant women who smoked or used cocaine. When a sound was played on the pregnant women's

bellies, an ultrasound showed that the babies opened their mouths in surprise.[99]

The probability of having twins is 31.2 per 1,000 live births, and to have triplet or higher order birth rate is 80.0 per 100,000 live births. The greatest number of babies born at once is 8, 6 boys and 2 girls.[100]

The process of ovulation[101]

When an **egg is mature**, it leaves the ovary, moves down the fallopian tube, and is ready to be fertilized. This is called ovulation. Every month or so, an egg will mature inside one of your ovaries. It has become thicker on the inside of the uterus to get ready for the fertilized egg. The lining of the uterus and blood will be shed if there is no conception, so periods happen when an unfertilized egg and the wall of the uterus gets released out.

Here some **interesting facts**:

- Ovulation can be affected by stress, illness, or disruption of normal routine
- Some women may experience some light blood or spotting during ovulation
- Implantation of a fertilized egg normally takes place 6-12 days after ovulation
- Each woman is born with millions of immature eggs that are awaiting ovulation to begin
- A menstrual period can occur even if ovulation has not occurred
- Ovulation can occur even if a menstrual period has not occurred
- Some women experience pain/aching near ovaries during ovulation called 'middle pain'

---

[99] Business Insider - https://www.insider.com/surprising-facts-about-pregnancy-2018-9 (Published in September 2018)

[100] Centers for Disease Control and Prevention - https://www.cdc.gov/nchs/fastats/multiple.htm (Reviewed in April 2023)

[101] American Pregnancy Association - https://americanpregnancy.org/getting-pregnant/infertility/understanding-ovulation (Accessed in May 2024)

- If an egg is not fertilized, it disintegrates and is absorbed into the uterine lining

From the first day of a woman's period to the first day of her next period, which is her monthly cycle. The standard length of a woman's cycle is between 28 and 32 days, but some women may have cycles that are much shorter or much longer. From the first day of the last menstrual period, most women ovulate between day 11 and day 21 of their cycle. Many people call this part of a woman's cycle the "fertile time" because having sex during this time makes it more likely that she will get pregnant. Ovulation can happen at different times during a cycle, and it might happen on a different day every month. It is important to keep track of your cycle, and luckily, there are a lot of free fertility charting tools and apps that can help women find their most fertile days.

Preconception health[102]

Preconception health refers to the health status during the childbearing years, or the years people can have a child. It's about what people can do right now to protect the health of a baby they might have later on.
The goal of preconception health is to help people get and stay healthy throughout their lives. Also, no one plans to get an unplanned pregnancy, but it does happen often. In the US, about half of all pregnancies are not expected.
Not just women, but also men should also take care of their health before getting pregnant. As a partner, it means helping and encouraging the lady's health.

[102] Centers for Disease Control and Prevention - https://www.cdc.gov/preconception/planning.html (Reviewed in February 2023)

Before you get pregnant, you should talk to your doctor about preconception health care. You and your doctor will talk about your health history and what you can do before you get pregnant to help avoid some birth defects:

- **Health Problems**: If you have any health problems, make sure they are under control and being treated. Sexually transmitted diseases (STDs), diabetes, thyroid disease, high blood pressure, and chronic diseases are a few of these.
- **Lifestyle**: Tell your doctor if you smoke, drink alcohol, or use certain drugs; if you live in a dangerous or cruel place; or if you work with or are near toxic substances. Counseling, treatment, and other types of support can be given to you by health care experts.
- Get to and stay at a healthy **weight**. Overweight or obese people are more likely to get a lot of dangerous conditions, including complications during pregnancy as well as heart disease, type 2 diabetes, and some types of cancer (endometrial, breast, and colon). Also, people who are too thin can have major health problems.
- **Medicines**: Almost all pregnant women will have to decide whether to take medicines before or during their pregnancy. When you start or stop taking drugs, talk to your doctor or nurse.
- **Vaccines**: Most vaccines are safe to get while pregnant, and some, like the flu shot and the Tdap (adult tetanus, diphtheria, and pertussis), are even suggested.
- Every Day, take 400 mg of **Folic Acid**, a type of vitamin B. Getting enough folic acid at least 1 month before and during pregnancy can help protect the baby's brain and spine from potential problems. You can get it from supplements and foods: broccoli, brussels sprouts, peas, chickpeas, kidney beans, and leafy greens like cabbage, kale, spring greens, and spinach are all good sources.
- Learn from your **family**'s health background. This can help you figure out what might affect your baby as an infant or child, or it

could affect your ability to get pregnant. It's possible that you don't know how your sister's heart problem or your cousin's sickle cell disease could affect your baby. Telling your doctor about this can be helpful. Your doctor may send you to genetic counseling based on the health background of your family. You might also need genetic counseling if you've had a lot of miscarriages, infant deaths, infertility, or if you had a genetic condition or birth defect during a previous pregnancy.

- Take care of your **mental health**. Mental health is how you think, feel, and act as you deal with life. You need to like your life and value yourself to be at your best.

If you want to have a baby or are just thinking about it, you can **start getting ready** for it right away. Health care and preconception health are all about things you can do before and after getting pregnant to improve your chances of having a healthy baby. It can take a few months for some people to get their bodies ready for pregnancy. It could take longer for some people.

Early signs of pregnancy[103]

What are the most common early signs of pregnancy?

- You missed your **period**. In the event that you are of sexual age and your period is late by a week or more, you may be pregnant. But this sign might be misleading if your period isn't regular.
- **Breasts** that hurt and swell up. As you get pregnant, changes in your hormones may make your breasts sore and sensitive. As your body gets used to the changes in hormones, the discomfort should go away after a few weeks.
- **Nausea**, with or without throwing up. It's common for morning sickness to start one month after becoming pregnant, however

[103] American Pregnancy Association - https://americanpregnancy.org/pregnancy-symptoms/early-signs-of-pregnancy (Accessed in May 2024)

it can happen at any time of the day or night. Some women feel sick earlier than others, and some never do.

- **Urinating** more often. You may need to go to the bathroom more often than normal, because during pregnancy, your body makes more blood, which makes your kidneys handle extra water that ends up in your bladder.
- You are **tired**. In the early stages of pregnancy, your body makes a lot of the hormone progesterone, which can make you feel sleepy.

You might have signs of pregnancy less than a week after getting pregnant, but some women say that for a few weeks, they didn't have any signs.

Reasons for infertility[104]

A little over 15% of couples have trouble getting pregnant. Many times, a couple is infertile if they can't have a baby after having sex without protection for at least 1 year, or for 6 months or more if she is over 35 years old.

Couples ages 29 to 33 whose reproductive systems are normally working have only a 20–25% chance of getting pregnant in any given month. By age 40, this chance drops to just 5%. Only 60% of couples who have been trying for 6 months will be able to get pregnant without medical help.

About 90% of the time, infertility is caused by one or more of these 3 things:

- Male factors, such as **sperm** production that is low or blockages
- **Egg** quality and number going down
- Problems in the **tubes**, like blockages in the fallopian tubes

There are **many factors** that can affect your ability to get pregnant. Some of these are age, food and nutrition, environment, weight, and health in general. Sometimes, all it takes is a little information, some

[104] American Pregnancy Association - https://americanpregnancy.org/resources/fertility-products-resource-guide (Accessed in May 2024)

patience, and some changes to how you live your life to make it much easier to get pregnant.

Several **thrombophilia** risk factors for early and late pregnancy loss were found. These include mutations that seem to affect fetal growth, especially in the first or second trimester. But right now, it's not recommended that women who have never had problems during pregnancy get tested regularly for thrombophilia problems. Because hereditary thrombophilia is so rare in the general population, previous studies on the subject often didn't have enough participants to find any useful results. And even though thrombophilia screening is safe and works, there is no treatment that has been shown to lower the rate of repeated pregnancy loss after screening.[105]

Menopause[106]

Due to **loss of ovarian follicular activity**, most women reach menopause when they stop having periods every month. This means that the ovaries stop putting out eggs that can be fertilized.

During woman's reproductive years, her periods become less regular and vary in length, but for most women around the world, menopause happens naturally between the ages of 45 and 55.

When a woman hasn't had her period for 12 months in a row and there isn't any other clear physiological or pathological reason, and no medical intervention has been made, this is defined as the **natural menopause**.

For some women, menopause starts earlier, before they turn 40. This **premature menopause** could be caused by genetic problems, autoimmune diseases, or something else that we don't know about yet.

---

[105] International Journal of Environmental Research and Public Health - https://www.ncbi.nlm.nih.gov/pmc/articles/PMC9779542 (Published in December 2022)

[106] World Health Organization - https://www.who.int/news-room/fact-sheets/detail/menopause (Published in October 2022)

There is no way to know for sure when a woman will go through menopause, but there are links between the age at menopause and some health, genetic, and social factors.
You can also go through menopause after surgery in which both ovaries are removed or after medical treatments that stop the ovaries from working, like radiation therapy or chemotherapy.
During perimenopause, it is still possible to get pregnant. It is suggested that you use birth control to avoid getting pregnant by accident until you have gone 12 months without having your period. Without fertility treatment that uses donor eggs or embryos that have already been frozen, getting pregnant after menopause is not possible.

The changes in hormones that happen during menopause can have an **impact** on your physical, mental, emotional, and social health. Menopause symptoms are very different for each woman, both during and after the change. Few or no signs show up for some, while in other cases symptoms can be very bad and make it hard to do daily things and enjoy life. Some women can have symptoms for years. During and after menopause, **you might experience**:

- Hot flashes and night sweats. A hot flush is a sudden feeling of heat in the face, neck, and chest that is often followed by flushing of the skin, perspiration (sweating), palpitations, and acute physical discomfort that can last for minutes.
- Changes in the regularity and flow of your menstrual cycle, ending with no periods at all.
- Dryness in the vaginal area, pain during sexual activity, and incontinence.
- Trouble sleeping or insomnia.
- Mood swings, depression, or anxiety.

The way your body looks and your chance of heart disease can also change. With a big drop in estrogen levels after menopause, women no longer have an advantage over men when it comes to heart disease. During menopause, the structures that support the pelvis can weaken, which raises the risk of pelvic organ prolapse. Loss of bone mass during menopause is also a big reason why more women get osteoporosis and break bones.

There are many hormonal and non-hormonal **treatments** that can help ease the symptoms of menopause. If you have symptoms that affect your health and well-being, you should talk to a health care provider about them so that you can find the best way to treat them, taking into account your medical background, values, and preferences.

It is important to remember that menopause is only one time in life. When a woman hits perimenopause, her health will mostly depend on her past health and reproductive history, as well as her lifestyle and the surroundings she lives in. During and after menopause, symptoms can make it hard to do things at work and in your personal life. As a woman ages, the changes that come with menopause will also affect her health. This is why **perimenopausal care** is so important for promoting healthy aging and a good quality of life.
In addition to being a bodily change, menopause can be a big change in a woman's life. Socially, a woman's menopause experience may be affected by gender roles, family, and sociocultural factors, such as how her culture views women getting older and the menopause transition.

Egg freezing[107]

Women can keep their fertility by freezing their eggs so they can try to have a family in the future. It involves getting eggs from the woman, freezing them, and then letting them thaw so that they can be used in fertility treatment.
Naturally, as a woman ages, her chances of getting pregnant decreases because the quality and amount of her eggs go down so individuals may try to maintain their fertility by freezing their eggs when they are still young and in their best health.

---

[107] Human Fertilisation and Embryology Authority - https://www.hfea.gov.uk/treatments/fertility-preservation/egg-freezing (Accessed in May 2024)

You might want to freeze your eggs if:

- You have a medical condition, like cancer, or need care for a medical condition that will make it hard for you to have children. Fertility may be preserved either by storing eggs, embryos, or a combination of both
- You're worried that your fertility is going down but aren't ready to have a child or haven't found the right partner
- You're at risk of injury or dying
- You're a woman transitioning to a man. You may want to keep your fertility alive before you start hormone therapy or have reconstructive surgery, since both methods can make you lose some or all of your fertility.

Contraception methods[108]

Many things must be evaluated by women, men, and couples at any point in their lives when picking the best way of birth control.

Intrauterine contraception, such as the Levonorgestrel Intrauterine system (LNG IUD) and the Copper T Intrauterine Device (IUD), is the most effective reversible method of birth control. They are small tools that look like the letter "T", and a doctor puts it inside the uterus. Every day, it sends out a small amount of progestin to keep you from getting pregnant. Based on the type of device, it can stay in your uterus for up to 3 to 10 years. Failure rate in normal use is 0.1% to 1.8%

Hormonal Methods are also pretty reliable; only about 4% to 7% of the time do they not work. This failure happens when some women may make an enzyme that breaks down birth control hormones in case they have a rare genetic version. This might help explain why the pill hasn't

[108] Centers for Disease Control and Prevention - https://www.cdc.gov/reproductivehealth/contraception/index.htm (Reviewed in May 2023)

worked for everyone and why some women who use it for birth control still get pregnant.[109]
Birth control pills can have side effects, just like any other medicine, but most of them go away after 2 or 3 months. Having sore breasts, feeling sick, or getting headaches are the most common side effects. Spots or bleeding between periods are also common, though only with progestin pills. It's fine for many women to take the pill. There are lots of different kinds of birth control, so you can choose from those. After 3 months of taking the pill, if you are still bothered by side effects, talk to your doctor about trying a different pill or a different way of birth control. You won't be safe from getting pregnant if you stop taking the pill and don't start a new method right away. A very small number of women who take the birth control pill have serious problems. Women who use combination pills or other forms of birth control that contain estrogen are a little more likely to have a few rare but dangerous problems than people who don't use birth control with hormones.[110]

Physical barriers, like condoms for both men and women, have a failure rate that runs from 13% to 21%. For both pregnancy and sexually transmitted diseases (STDs), condoms are great. If you follow the directions and use them every time you have oral, anal, or vaginal sex, there's almost no chance of getting or passing an STD, and they will stop you from getting pregnant 98% of the time.
In other words, you have to wear it the whole time. Before you touch your genital to someone else's, make sure the condom is on correctly. Wearing two condoms at once is not a good idea, and neither is putting one on your penis and another internal condom. Condoms are meant to be used by themselves, and using two of them together may make them more likely to tear. The condom should be ready to roll on with the rim facing outward, making it look like a small hat, and it should also be easy to unroll. It can be rolled up a bit to make sure it's the right way out

---

[109] Obstetrics and Gynecology - https://journals.lww.com/greenjournal/abstract/2019/04000/influence_of_genetic_variants_on_steady_state.27.aspx (Published in April 2019)
[110] Planned Parenthood - https://www.plannedparenthood.org/learn/birth-control/birth-control-pill/what-are-the-disadvantages-of-the-pill (Accessed in May 2024)

before putting it on. If you put on a condom backwards by accident, DO NOT turn it over and use it again; get a new one. Put the condom on your penis and pinch the tip of it, leaving some room at the top to gather the semen (cum). Before you roll it on, you can put a few drops of water-based or silicone lube in the condom's tip, and after putting the condom, you can also add more lube to the outside of it. Lubes that are water-based or made of silicone can make sex feel even better and keep condoms from breaking. Things like Vaseline, lotion, baby oil, butter, and cooking oils all have oil in them, so don't use them with rubber condoms, because latex condoms can break if they get oil on them. Don't store your condoms in direct sunlight or somewhere sharp; instead, keep them somewhere cool and dry. Don’t keep them in the bathroom, your bag, or your car for more than 1 month, since too much heat and moisture can damage condoms over time. Check the date on the condoms' wrapper or box to make sure they are still good. When you're done ejaculating (cum), grab the condom's edge and pull your penis away from your partner, before your penis gets soft. That way, the condom won't get too loose and let semen out.[111]

Other contraceptives, but that aren't very reliable, are:

- **Fertility Awareness-Based methods**: If you have a regular period, you have at least 9 fertile days every month. If you don't want to get pregnant, you either don't have sex on days when you could get pregnant or use those days birth control with barrier methods. Failure rates range from 2% to 23%.
- **Pulling out**, also called "withdrawal": it means taking the penis out of the vagina before ejaculation. If you want the pull-out method to work, you should use it with another kind of birth control. Pre-ejaculate, which is also called pre-cum, is a fluid that comes out of the penis when it's excited. It usually happens right before ejaculation. The fluid naturally smooths things out

[111] Planned Parenthood - https://www.plannedparenthood.org/learn/birth-control/condom (Accessed in May 2024)

during sex, and some of it can even contain live sperm. Range of failure rates is 22%.[112]

An emergency method of birth control is NOT a normal way to avoid pregnancy. Emergency birth control can be used if there was no birth control during sex or if the way of birth control didn't 5, like if a condom broke.

- **Copper IUD**—Women can get the copper T IUD put in up to five days after having sex without protection.
- **Emergency birth control pills** that women can take up to 5 days after having sex without protection. However, the earlier they are taken, the better they will work.

Permanent birth control is a very safe option, and it refers to the sterilization:

- **Tubal ligation** or "tying tubes", when a woman's fallopian tubes can be closed or tied so that sperm and eggs can't meet and fertilize each other. Failure rate is 0.5%.
- Men can be sterilized by having a **vasectomy**, which stops their sperm from getting to their penis. This way, their ejaculate never has any sperm in it. Failure rate is 0.15%.

Sexual dysfunction[113]

Sexual dysfunction, or sexual disorder, means that you are having trouble having sex or liking it, and this makes you feel bad. Having sex can be good for your health and happiness, so it can be hard to deal with sexual dysfunction on a mental and physical level. A lot of people have sexual problems, and most of the time, they can be helped.

---

[112] Planned Parenthood - https://www.plannedparenthood.org/learn/birth-control/withdrawal-pull-out-method/how-effective-is-withdrawal-method-pulling-out (Accessed in May 2024)

[113] Planned Parenthood - https://www.plannedparenthood.org/learn/sex-pleasure-and-sexual-dysfunction/sexual-dysfunction (Accessed in May 2024)

Some examples of sexual problems are:

- **Hypoactive Sexual Desire Disorder (HSDD)**: This is when you are not interested in having sex and it makes you feel bad. For people with HSDD, sexual thoughts and fantasies are very rare. They also don't react to their partner's sexual signals or hints, lose the desire for sex while having it, or don't want it at all.
- **Erectile Dysfunction**: If your penis can't get hard enough to have sex or stay hard enough to finish having sex. An erection is something that a lot of men have trouble with at some point in their lives. Getting older is one of many things that can make it hard to get or keep an erection, but this can happen to anyone, not just older people.
- **Orgasm Disorder**: This is when you don't have orgasms, it takes a long time for you to orgasm, you don't have orgasms as often as you'd like, or they're not as strong as you'd like. Your hormones, physical health, emotions, experiences, believes, lifestyle, and relationships are just a few of the things that affect your orgasm.
- **Vulvodynia**: This is when you have pain in your vulva that isn't caused by an illness or another health issue and lasts for 3 months or more. Pain and irritability like burning, stinging, rawness, aching, soreness, throbbing, and swelling are signs of vulvodynia. This could affect just one part of your vulva or the whole structure. The signs of vulvodynia can be present all the time or only sometimes. Symptoms may happen at random or only when your vulva is touched or something goes inside your vagina. Having sex, using a tampon, getting a pelvic exam, wearing tight pants, or sitting for a long time are all things that can cause or make vulvodynia symptoms worse. Vulvodynia doesn't always have a clear cause, it's likely caused by a lot of different things acting together.
- **Premature Ejaculation**: This is when you ejaculate (cum) before you want to, generally before your partner has an orgasm. If it happens once in a while, don't worry about it, but if it happens more than half of the time you try to have sex, you might want to talk to a doctor about it. There is no clear cause for premature

ejaculation, but it is most likely psychological or mental. People who are nervous about their sexual performance or who aren't used to having sex, like people who have never had sex before, are more likely to ejaculate before they're ready.

Sexual problems can be **caused** by many things, and for many people, more than one, such as stress, fear and anxiety about sex, using drugs or alcohol, hormone levels, mental health problems (like depression), problems in your relationship, certain medicines and treatments, menopause, being pregnant, breastfeeding, giving birth, or medical problems like cancer, diabetes, heart problems, multiple sclerosis, or bladder problems.
How sexual problems are treated depends on what caused them. That's why talking to a doctor can help you figure out what's wrong and get the help you need.

Kids are small humans?[114-115]

Before birth and in the first 2 years of life, the brain grows the fastest. At this time, it's especially **important** to take care of the health by eating well and getting enough rest. 80% of the structure of the brain forms between the ages of 0 and 3, and 90% until age 5.
Babies talk by reacting to even the smallest sounds, movements, and even the smell of the person caring for them. The caregiver and the baby's interaction turn into a dance when the caretaker answers back. When someone holds, loves, and makes the baby feel safe, the baby "attaches" to that person, and this bond or link lasts a lifetime.[116]
Kids love to try new things and learn new skills all the time. For them to be able to play and learn without getting hurt, the place where they are

[114] World Health Organization - https://www.who.int/health-topics/child-health (Accessed in May 2024)
[115] CNN - https://edition.cnn.com/2023/03/29/health/us-children-gun-deaths-dg/index.html (Updated in March 2023)
[116] UNICEF - https://www.unicef.org/turkiye/en/stories/10-facts-about-early-childhood-development-you-need-know (Published in November 2015)

needs to be clean, safe, and well-guarded. There are more than 200 million kids younger than 5 who are not developing as they should be.

More than a quarter of American teens and young adults have been through a major **traumatic event** by the time they are 16, and many kids go through even more than one traumatic event. Child abuse and neglect, major accidents, disasters, terrorism, and experiencing or seeing violence in neighborhoods, schools, and homes, treatment for a life-threatening illness are all common causes of trauma. The chance of a child getting traumatic stress after a disaster or traumatic event is high. Post-Traumatic Stress Disorder (PTSD), depression, or anxiety problems affect about one-quarter of people who have been victims or witnesses of violence.[117]

How are children different from adults?[118]

Children's **bodies** are different from adults' bodies, and there is a greater possibility that they will become ill or badly wounded.
The amount of air that they take in per pound of body weight is greater than what adults take in.
Their skin is thinner, and they have a greater amount of it per pound of body weight, which results in a higher surface-to-mass ratio.
Then, as a result of having a lower fluid content in their bodies, children are more susceptible to experiencing the effects of fluid loss, such as dehydration and blood loss.
They have also a greater propensity to shed an excessive amount of body heat.
Their time spent outside and on the ground is significantly increased, and in addition to this, children are more likely than adults to put their hands in their mouths.

---

[117] National Child Traumatic Stress Network - http://melissainstitute.org/documents/ChildTraumaBasicFacts.pdf (Accessed in May 2024)
[118] Centers for Disease Control and Prevention - https://www.cdc.gov/childrenindisasters/differences.html (Reviewed in September 2020)

Children also need help from adults in case of an **emergency**.
First, they do not have a complete understanding of how to preserve their own safety.
Younger toddlers and teenagers may draw their signals from the actions and behaviors of others.
Then, in case an emergency happens, it is possible for children to experience freezing, crying, or screaming, and they might not be able to articulate the information that causes them pain or annoyance.
When they are in the presence of their parents or other caregivers, they have a greater chance of receiving the care that they require, since it is required by law for an adult to make decisions regarding a child's medical care.
There is a lack of information regarding the ways in which some diseases and medications have an effect on youngsters. At times, individuals will be required to make judgments based on the information that they have available to them.

Finally, mental **stress** from a disaster can be harder on children. As a result, they have a diminished sense of control, a restricted understanding of the circumstance, and they are less likely to have had the opportunity to recover from challenging situations.

Effective parenting practices[119]

The act of parenting can take various forms, yet there are certain parenting methods that are effective across a wide range of families and environments. The following are the most **important ways** in which parents may support the healthy development of their children:

- Following the child’s lead and responding in a predictable way
- Showing warmth and sensitivity
- Having routines and household rules
- Sharing books and talking with children
- Supporting health and safety
- Using appropriate discipline without harshness

[119] Centers for Disease Control and Prevention - https://www.cdc.gov/ncbddd/childdevelopment/features/parenting-matters.html (Reviewed in February 2023)

Top causes of deaths for children

It is of the utmost significance to prioritize the protection and enhancement of the health of children. Over the course of the last few decades, we have witnessed significant **advancements** concerning the improvement of health and the reduction of the death rate among young children. The number of children who passed away globally before the age of 5 was cut in half between the years 2000 and 2017, and the number of moms and children who are still alive today is higher than it has ever been. These are just two of the promising facts.
Despite this, there is still a significant amount of work to be done in order to better enhance the health outcomes for children. There is a dual mission that the world must fulfill. Greater than 50% of the deaths that occur in children are the result of illnesses that are easily preventable or treatable, provided that children have access to medical care and improvements in their quality of life. At the same time, it is essential to provide children with a secure environment in which they can flourish. This environment should include a healthy and nutritious diet, protection from potential dangers, and access to chances for learning and development. In order to construct a more favorable future, one of the most essential actions that a society can take is to make investments in children.

A child's odds of survival are vastly different in different parts of the **world**, with countries with low and moderate incomes being disproportionately affected because of these discrepancies. Child mortality rates in Sub-Saharan Africa are among the highest in the world, with some regions having rates that are 15 times higher than those in nations with high incomes. Infections of the respiratory system, diseases that cause diarrhea, measles, malaria, malnutrition are among the top causes of death among children. Vaccination, sufficient home care, access to health care services, increased rates of breastfeeding, and improved nutrition are all practices that can help avoid a significant number of deaths that occur among children. Nevertheless, most of the interventions that could save lives are completely out of reach for the poorest people in the world.

Now, double clicking on the high-income countries, the **top 5** causes of deaths for children ages 1 to 18, as a percentage of all causes in US in 2021:

- Firearms: 19%
- Traffic accident: 16%
- Cancer: 8%
- Poisoning: 7%
- Suffocation: 6%

Firearms

Since 2020, firearms have surpassed automobile accidents as the main cause of death among children and adolescents in the United States.
According to the Wonder database maintained by the Centers for Disease Control and Prevention, firearms were responsible for roughly 19% of all deaths that occurred among children aged 1 to 18 in the year 2021, which numbered over 3,600 children lost their lives as a result of gun-related incidents. This means that about 5 children are lost for every 100,000 in the United States, according to this estimate. Firearms are not among the top 4 causes of children death in any other comparable country.
According to the findings of a new study published in JAMA, the rise in child and teen mortality that occurred during the COVID-19 pandemic was not caused by deaths caused by the COVID-19 virus but rather by fatal injuries, and more specifically nearly half of the rise in mortality that occurred in the year 2020 was attributed to firearms.

Traffic accident[120]

As a result of automobile accidents, thousands of young children are either killed or injured every year. When used correctly, automobile safety seats contribute to the protection of children. On the other hand,

---

[120] CNN - https://edition.cnn.com/2018/01/29/health/newborn-mistakes-parents/index.html (Published in January 2018)

many parents find this to be overwhelming because there are so many different seats available on the market.
When it came to installing their car seats or placing their newborns in those seats, 91% of the parents made severe mistakes according to a 2016 study published in the Journal of Pediatrics and that included roughly 300 families. 86% of those errors affected the positioning of the baby in the seat, and the majority of those errors were considered "critical" because they raised the likelihood that the kid would sustain an injury in the event of an accident. Over half of the families had children who were older, which ought to have provided them with practice for this task.[121]
Parents should take care to ensure that their newborn child's head does not fall forward, as this could potentially impede the infant's ability to breathe. In order to accomplish this, the seat must be installed at the appropriate angle to ensure that the baby's feet remain elevated. Additionally, the torso must be reclined so that the infant can move her head to the side and breathe normally. Using a tightly rolled receiving blanket on both sides of the baby or using the newborn insert that is manufactured for that particular brand of car seat is recommended by the American Academy of Pediatrics in the event that the baby slouches down or to the side while seated in the car seat. It is important to note that you should not mix and match with other manufacturers. It is important to avoid placing a blanket or roll over the top of the baby's head, as well as placing padding under the youngster.[122]

---

[121] Journal of Pediatrics - https://www.jpeds.com/article/S0022-3476(15)01459-6/fulltext (Published in December 2015)
[122] American Academy of Pediatrics - https://www.healthychildren.org/English/safety-prevention/on-the-go/Pages/Car-Safety-Seats-Information-for-Families.aspx (Updated in January 2023)

Poisoning[123]

There are occasions when children engage in activities that they most likely ought not to. Things that are commonly found in the home, such as cleaning supplies and personal care goods, have the potential to be hazardous to children.

In order to decrease the risk of poisoning in children, the Centers for Disease Control and Prevention and the American Academy of Pediatrics have provided the following **recommendations**:

- It is important to ensure that youngsters are unable to see or access certain substances, such as pesticides, paints and varnishes, cleaning and laundry products, and medicines. Whenever it is feasible, keep these items hidden away.
- It is important to ensure that these goods are always stored in their original containers, because this will reduce the likelihood that they may be accidentally consumed.
- If there are young children in the house, you should consider the traditional liquid and powder detergents; even though laundry and dishwasher detergent pods can be convenient. Simply said, the pods have an appearance that is too similar to that of candy.
- All drugs should be equipped with safety caps.
- Get rid of any medicines or cleaning goods that are outdated or have not been used. The less of them there are, the fewer the risk.
- You should only purchase nicotine refills in safety containers if you use electronic cigarettes, and you should store them out of sight and out of reach. Using nicotine can be quite hazardous for children.
- Know which of the electronic items in your home are powered by button cell batteries, and make sure that youngsters cannot access them. Avoid purchasing books or toys for children that contain these batteries; the danger is not worth taking.

---

[123] Harvard Health Publishing - https://www.health.harvard.edu/blog/how-to-prevent-poisonings-in-children-and-what-to-do-if-they-happen-2019031916230 (Published in March 2019)

- Ensure that you are familiar with all of the different kinds of plants that you have in your home or yard. In the event that any of them are poisonous, you should either keep your child away from them or, even better, get rid of them.

What to do **if someone gets poisoned** or if you think he/she might have:

- Call the emergency number right away if the child is having trouble breathing, is unconscious, or has what you think might be a major injury.
- If the child swallowed poison, have them spit out what they didn't swallow. Do not make them throw up with syrup of ipecac or anything else. Call an emergency number or take your child to a nearby health center if they show any of these signs. If your child doesn't seem sick, call the poison control center across the country (in the US, that number is 1-800-222-1222), having the poison container with you. Be ready to tell them how much your child took, or your best guess. You should save the Poison Control Center's number in your phone and put it somewhere visible in your home.
- If it gets on the kid's skin, take off all of your clothes and run water over the area for 15 minutes. You should also call the poison center at the same time.
- If anything gets in the eyes, keep your eyes open and run room-temperature water over the inside corner of your eye for 15 minutes. As you flush the eyes, call the poison center or the emergency number if a lot got into the eyes or the child is in a lot of pain, but do not stop flushing.

Suffocation[124]

Babies can't get out of a position where they can't breathe because of their weakness, and they can last a few minutes before they die of suffocation. Kids younger than 5 are most likely to be victims in these stories.

---

[124] Child Accident Prevention Trust - https://capt.org.uk/suffocation-prevention (Accessed in September 2023)

To lower this chance, take a look at these **tips**:

- **Safe places** to sleep: a cot of their own is the safest place for them to sleep. A lot of people sleep with their babies, especially in the first few months when they wake up all the time. Some babies have been suffocated by their parents by mistake, which is very sad. Not often, but it is very dangerous if the person sleeping with the baby has been drinking or using drugs, is very tired, or smokes, or if the baby was born before 37 weeks or weighed less than 2.5 kg.
- **Bedding**: tiny babies aren't strong enough to pull blankets away from their faces, so if they get stuck under the covers, they can sometimes asphyxiate. Place babies at the bottom of the crib so their feet touch the end, and this will keep them from moving around. Duvets and quilts should not be used with babies younger than 12 months because they can't move the clothing away from their faces. Instead, use blankets or a lightweight sleeping bag that doesn't have a hood and is the right size so the baby can't get inside it. With babies younger than 12 months, you should never use a pillow.
- **Snacks**: for babies younger than 6 months, it's normal for them to grab things and pull them to their mouths. Nappy snacks are very thin, so they can easily stick to a baby's face as it breathes in. Sadly, some babies have died of suffocation after being able to reach and grab a nappy sack. To keep babies safe, we say keep nappy bags out of their reach and never put them in a cot, pram, or buggy.
- **Niches**: some babies can move around a lot, even though they can't walk or crawl yet. They will move around and wiggle, roll, and squirm, and their little heads can get stuck in tight spaces. Make sure there is no more than 4 cm of space between their mattress and the cot bars to keep them safe.
- **Sofas**: it can be dangerous to put a baby to sleep on a sofa, even though it's often handy to do so. A lot of chairs have big gaps between the cushions. All of these can choke your baby if they get stuck.

- **Slings**: The baby is most at risk when they are in a C-shape, with their chin on their chest, because this can make it hard for them to breathe. These kids are more likely to suffocate if they were born early, had a low birth weight, are having trouble breathing, or have a cold. If you use a sling, follow the TICKS advice: keep your baby Tight, In view, Close enough to kiss, Keep their chin off their chest, and Supported back.
- **Plastic bags**: keep in mind that toddlers can get to a lot of things they shouldn't, like plastic bags. One easy way to keep them safe is to tie a knot near the top of the bag: if your kid can't open the bag, he won't be able to choke! Many new goods and appliances, especially big ones, come with plastic sheets that seal and protect them. If you don't throw them away right away, these sheets can also be dangerous, so keep this kind of thing out of your child's reach.
- Kids **3 to 5 years old**: Now that they are this old, kids can sleep with duvets and blankets. Because they are curious and want to play, there is still a small chance that they will suffocate.

Aging and personal care

"Age is inevitable. Aging isn't"
Marv Levy (former American football coach and executive)

At the biological level, getting older is caused by a buildup of different kinds of molecule and cellular damage over time. This slowly lowers your physical and mental abilities, making you more likely to get sick and eventually to die. These changes don't happen in a straight line over time, and they have little to do with how old someone is in years. The diversity seen in older age is not random.

Some changes that come with getting older are normal, like graying hair. Some other common health problems in older people are hearing loss,

cataracts, refractive errors, back and neck pain, osteoarthritis, diabetes, depression, and dementia.
As people get older, they also start to experience a number of complicated health conditions known as **geriatric syndromes**. These problems usually have more than one cause, and some examples are frailty, urinary incontinence, falls, delirium, and pressure ulcers.

There is no one type of older person. Some 80-year-olds are mentally and physically as sharp as many 30-year-olds, while some others start to lose a lot of their abilities at much younger ages.
A big part of it has to do with people's physical and social **environments** and how they affect their health and the chances they have. People's relationships with their surroundings are skewed by factors like their race, gender, or the family they were born into. This can cause health disparities.
People often think that older people are weak, needy, and a drag on society. People who work in public health and society as a whole need to deal with these and other ageist views that can lead to discrimination, change how policies are made, and limit older people's chances to age in a healthy way.
In direct and indirect ways, globalization, new technologies (like those used in transportation and communication), movement, living in cities, and changes in gender roles are all affecting the lives of older people.[125]

---

[125] World Health Organization - https://www.who.int/news-room/fact-sheets/detail/ageing-and-health (Published in October 2022)

Our skin

Skin is our largest organ—adults carry some 8 pounds (3.6 kilograms) and 22 square feet (2 square meters) of it.[126]
About 30,000 to 40,000 dead skin cells are peeled off the top of our skin every minute, even though you can't see it, and that's nearly 9 pounds (4 kg) of cells every year! Your epidermis is always making new skin cells, which rise to the surface to take the place of the old ones. On your skin's surface, 95% of the cells make new skin cells.[127]

10 ways to reduce premature skin aging[128]

It's normal for skin to get thinner and drier as people age, and lines and other signs of aging increase. Sometimes the things around you and the way you live can make your face age faster than it should, so dermatologists say to follow these simple **tips** to keep your face from aging too quickly:

1. Keep your face out of the **sun**. Sun protection is important whether you're going to the beach or doing some duties. To protect your face, find shade, wear clothes that block the sun, and use broad-spectrum sunscreen with an SPF of 30 or higher that is water-resistant. The sunscreen should be put on all skin that isn't hidden by clothes every day. For better defense, look for clothes that have a sticker that says "UPF" (Ultraviolet Protection Factor).
2. Use **self-tanner** instead of going out and getting one. Getting a tan makes your face age faster than it should. And this is true whether you get your tan in the sun, a tanning bed, or with

---

[126] Better Health - https://www.betterhealth.vic.gov.au/health/conditionsandtreatments/skin (Reviewed in October 2023)
[127] Kids Health - https://kidshealth.org/en/kids/skin.html (Reviewed in January 2023)
[128] American Academy of Dermatology Association - https://www.aad.org/public/everyday-care/skin-care-secrets/anti-aging/reduce-premature-aging-skin (Updated in February 2021)

some tool. All of them give off UV rays that are bad for you and make your skin age faster.

3. Don't **smoke** anymore. When you smoke, your face ages a lot faster. It makes your skin look dull and shallow and gives you wrinkles.
4. Don't make the same **facial gestures** over and over. When you make a face expression, the muscles below get tight, and if you tighten the same muscles over and over for years, the lines will stay there. Sunglasses can help get rid of lines that come from squinting.
5. Make sure you eat a healthy, varied **diet**. A few studies have shown that eating a lot of fresh fruits and veggies may help protect against damage that causes skin to age faster. A diet high in sugar and other refined carbohydrates may also speed up the aging process.
6. Don't **drink** as much. Alcohol is rough on the skin, since it makes the skin dry and, over time, damages the face.
7. **Work out** most days a week.
8. **Wash** your face properly: read the next chapter on this point.
9. Use **lotion** on your face every day. Moisturizer keeps water in our skin, which makes look younger. When putting cream around your eyes, be careful not to pull too hard on the skin there.
10. Stop using **skin care products** that burn or sting your skin. This means that there is something wrong with this product on your skin irritating it.

You might want to see a doctor if the signs of aging skin bother you. Many people are getting younger-looking skin thanks to new treatments and less invasive processes that get rid of wrinkles, tighten skin, and make the skin look better.

Face washing 101[129]

What you do when you wash your face can change how you look. Derms have given you these tips to help you keep your face looking healthy:

- Use a cleaner that is gentle, won't scratch, and doesn't have alcohol in it. You can get rid of dirt, makeup, and other things that are bad for your skin by washing gently.
- Wet your face with tepid water, and then use your fingers to put on the cleanser. Anything other than your fingers can irritate your skin, like a washcloth or a mesh sponge.
- Don't scrub your skin because it will irritate it.
- Use tepid water to rinse, and then dry with a soft towel.
- Only wash twice a day, once in the morning, once at night, and again right after you sweat a lot. The skin gets irritated by sweat, especially when a hat or helmet is on.

Watch the respective video by American Academy of Dermatology:
https://youtu.be/AeXsfB2ud-o?si=ONuxsk4p7kXBUMzv

[129] American Academy of Dermatology Association - https://www.aad.org/public/everyday-care/skin-care-basics/care/face-washing-101 (Accessed in May 2024)

How to select anti-aging skin care products[130, 131]

It can be hit or miss when you're shopping for anti-aging skin care products. It can be hard to decide which goods to buy when there are so many to pick from. You can feel more confident about shopping after reading these **tips**:

- Put on sunscreen and lotion first. Dermatologists all agree that moisturizer and sunscreen are the best anti-aging items you can buy. These can make a real difference if you use them every day. It's fine to use a lotion with sunscreen.
- Choose sunscreen that has all of the following when you go shopping: broad spectrum, at least SPF 30, and Resistance to water
- A lotion that fights aging can help get rid of fine lines. Because it works so well, moisturizer is often the secret ingredient in goods that fight aging.
- Take care of your main skin-aging worry. Allow sunscreen and lotion a few weeks to do their job, and after that, check out your face. Is there still an old age sign that worries you?
- If you only worry about one thing, like lines or dark spots, you'll get the best results. You should look for a solution that addresses specifically this issue. This is because of two things: using more than one anti-aging product in a few days or weeks can irritate the skin and make you look older; then, each product can only treat a few signs of age.
- Get a product that is made for the type of skin you have. Say, if your skin is oily, choose a moisturizer that is made for greasy skin, while the label should say "sensitive skin" if you have delicate skin.

---

[130] American Academy of Dermatology Association - https://www.aad.org/public/everyday-care/skin-care-secrets/anti-aging/selecting-anti-aging-products (Accessed in May 2024)

[131] American Academy of Dermatology Association - https://www.aad.org/public/everyday-care/skin-care-secrets/anti-aging/maximize-anti-aging-products (Accessed in May 2024)

- Please read the labels and choose a product that has all of the following: hypoallergenic means that the product may still cause an allergic response, but the chance of it happening is lower; non-comedogenic or non-acnegenic means that it does not cause acne; and there is a consumer hotline that you can call for questions.
- Pick an item that is in your price range. We all tend to believe that the more expensive something is, the better it works. Anti-aging goods that work come in a wide range of prices.
- Begin with one item. Before putting it on your face or hands, test the product first, because products that claim to be safe can still make your skin react. Put a little of the product on the inside of your wrist to test it, twice every day for 5 days and then if your skin doesn't itch, turn red, or react in any other way, you can put it on your face and other skin.
- Allow the product to do its job. In a few days, a lotion can smooth out fine lines, but most products need at least 6 weeks to fully work and even it may take up to 3 months sometimes. Wait a little while and let the product do its thing.
- Keep using it if you want to keep seeing results. Once a thing starts to work, most people stop using it.
- Don't set unrealistic goals. Too many claims are too good to be true, like saying you'll look 10 years younger overnight or that you'll quickly lose all signs of age. Keep in mind that anti-aging skin care items only work slightly better than placebo. It's not possible for a cream to work like a facelift.

How well your skin care products work depends on the order in which you use them. Dermatologists say that the following is the **best way to apply** them[132]:

1. Wash your face.

---

[132] American Academy of Dermatology Association - https://www.aad.org/public/everyday-care/skin-care-basics/care/apply-skin-care-certain-order(Accessed in May 2024)

2. If you are using medicine or other treatment on your skin, you should apply this right after cleansing.
3. When applying any cream around your eyes, use your ring finger, because it is the weakest finger and will not pull too hard on this delicate skin.
4. Apply moisturizer and/or sunscreen.
5. Apply makeup, if desired.

Sunburns[133]

If you don't wear sunscreen and clothes that protect your skin from the sun, you could get burned. If you want to help your skin heal and feel better, you should treat sunburn as soon as you notice it. Getting out of the sun and going inside is the first thing you should do.
Once you're inside, these tips can **help ease the pain**:

- Take cool showers or baths to ease the pain. Let a little water stay on your skin after you pat yourself dry after getting out of the tub or shower. After that, put on a moisturizer to help your skin hold on to the water, helping to make it less dry.
- Drink more water. The skin's surface pulls fluid away from the rest of the body when it gets burned. When you're burnt, drinking extra water can help you stay hydrated.
- To help sunburned skin feel better, use a lotion with aloe vera or soy in it. There is hydrocortisone cream that you can buy without a prescription that you might want to use on an area that hurts a lot. If you get a sunburn, don't use "-caine" products (i.e., benzocaine) to treat it. These can irritate the skin or cause an allergic response. You might want to take aspirin or ibuprofen to help lessen any pain, redness, and swelling.
- If you get blisters on your skin, let them heal. This means that you have a second-degree sunburn. You shouldn't pop the

[133] American Academy of Dermatology Association - https://www.aad.org/public/everyday-care/injured-skin/burns/treat-sunburn (Accessed in May 2024)

blisters because they form to help your skin heal and keep you from getting an infection.

- When you're outside, cover your face with clothes. Fabrics that are tightly woven work best. It should not let any light through when you hold it up to a bright light.

Age spots[134]

Age spots, which are also known as liver spots or solar lentigo, are groups of **pigments** that form on the skin from too much time in the sun. In the same way that a scar forms after a cut, pigment builds up after an injury. The color builds up in places where skin is damaged from being too thin having had too much sun, being caused by bruises that leave behind blood-colored skin. People older than 55 are most likely to have them. People often get the spots on their hands, but they can be almost anywhere, especially on areas that get a lot of sun, like the face, back, arms, feet, and shoulders.

You can lower your **risk** of getting age spots by spending less time in the sun. The main thing that affects how your skin will look later on is how much sun you get before you turn 20. Keeping out of the sun can help keep age spots from getting bigger or darker if you already have them.

Age spots might be a sign that you're past your prime, but you might be able to get rid of them.
There are 2 **ways to get rid** of age spots:

- **Lotions** and creams: they require discipline. A cream or oil needs to be used once or twice a day for weeks or months before it starts to work. There are many products on the market that promise to get rid of age spots, and you can buy a lot of them without a prescription.

---

[134] American Academy of Dermatology Association - https://www.aad.org/public/cosmetic/age-spots-marks/get-rid-spots (Published September 2021)

- **Procedures**, such as chemical peels and laser therapy, tend to work faster. Also, procedures are more likely to cause side effects and cost more.

It's important to know that age spots can come back no matter what care you take. You can avoid this by keeping your skin out of the sun.

Scars signs[135]

As soon as your skin gets injured, your body starts to heal it, and later a scar may form. This is a normal part of the process.
How a scar looks often depends on **how well the wound heals**. Surgery scars and scars over joints like the knees and elbows are hard to avoid. However, scars from small cuts and scrapes can be less noticeable if the wound is treated properly at home.

Here are some **tips** from dermatologists on how to make scars look less eye-catching:

- Always keep clean a cut, scrape, or other skin wound that you have. Wash the area gently with water and gentle soap to get rid of germs and dirt.
- Use petroleum jelly to keep the wound wet to help the skin heal. Putting petroleum jelly on the cut keeps it from drying out and making a scab, since wounds that have scabs take longer to heal. Also, this will keep a scar from getting too big, thick, or itchy. Antibacterial creams are not needed as long as the wound is cleaned every day.
- After you clean the area and put on petroleum jelly or a similar cream, put an adhesive bandage over the skin. Hydrogel or silicone gel sheets might help with big cuts, scrapes, sores, burns, or swelling.
- Change the wrap every day while the wound heals to keep it clean. If your skin is sensitive to glue, use paper tape on a cotton

[135] American Academy of Dermatology Association - https://www.aad.org/public/everyday-care/injured-skin/burns/wound-care-minimize-scars (Accessed in May 2024)

pad that doesn't stick. When you need to change silicone gel or hydrogel sheets, read, and follow the directions on the box.

- If you need stitches, do what your doctor tells you about how to take care of the wound and when to have the stitches taken out.
- After the cut has healed, put sunscreen on it. Keeping out of the sun may help the scar fade faster and lessen any red or brown spots that are there. Always use a broad-spectrum sunscreen with at least 30 SPF, and make sure you reapply it often.

What to know about tattoos[136]

Dermatologists are being asked by more and more people to give them skin care tips that will help tattoos look their best. Here are some tips on **how to keep skin with tattoos healthy** and glowing:

- If the skin with the tattoo feels dry, put on a lotion or cream that contains water. Creams made from petroleum, like petroleum jelly, can fade the ink.
- Keep the sun off of your tattoo, since a lot of UV light can fade some tattoo colors. Apply a broad-spectrum, water-resistant sunscreen with an SPF of 30 or more to your tattoo before going out in the sun to protect it. Apply the sunscreen 15 minutes before you go outside and reapply at least every 2 hours.
- Don't use sunlamps or tanning beds. These devices may also fade tattoo ink and raise your risk of getting skin cancer. In some people, the UV light may also react with the tattoo ink, which can be painful.
- Talk to a doctor if your skin reacts or changes in any way after getting a tattoo. The ink in a tattoo might not be good for your skin, and this could happen right away or years later after getting a tattoo. A change could also mean you have a skin disease, so a dermatologist can figure out what's wrong and fix it.

---

[136] American Academy of Dermatology Association - https://www.aad.org/public/everyday-care/skin-care-basics/tattoos/caring-for-tattooed-skin (Accessed in May 2024)

- If you want a new tattoo, think about getting it on skin that doesn't have any moles on it. It might be harder to spot the first signs of skin cancer if you have a tattoo on them. Skin cancer, even the most dangerous kind, melanoma, can be very easily treated if found early.

Hair loss as aging process[137]

We lose about 50 to 100 hairs every day, and most of the time we don't even notice.
There are **types** of hair loss that are permanents, like male and female pattern baldness, which often runs in the family, and there are other types of hair loss that may only be temporary. They can be brought on by being sick, stressed, getting treatment for cancer, losing weight, or not getting enough iron. If the doctor looks at your hair, they might be able to tell you what's making you lose it.

Hereditary hair loss is the most common cause in the world, and it can happen to both men and women. It's called androgenic alopecia in the medical world, independent of the person's gender. No matter what you call it, it means that you have genes that make your hair follicles (the holes in your skin where hair grows) get smaller and smaller until they stop growing hair altogether. They can start shrinking in your teens, but most of the time they don't do it until much later in life.
On the other hand, most people lose some hair as they get older because hair growth slows down. Hair cells stop making hair at some point, which makes scalp hair loss happen. The color of your hair starts to fade too.
If your hair loss is caused by a medical condition, it will generally stop or grow back after you get better.

If your hair loss is making you unhappy, there are some things you can try, but no **treatment** is 100% guaranteed to work.

---

[137] National Health Service - https://www.nhs.uk/conditions/hair-loss/ (Reviewed in February 2021)

Talk to your doctor about how your hair loss is affecting your health and ask about solutions.

These medicines can be pricey and don't always work for everyone, and they also only work as long as they're used.

A hair transfer is a surgery that moves hair from one place to another where it is thin or bald.

It's a big choice to get a hair transplant, so learn as much as you can about what's going to happen. The cost of a hair transplant can range from $1,000 to $30,000, and it depends on how much hair you've lost, the type of procedure you get, and how good the clinic and staff are. People who have lifelong baldness, like the kind that runs in families, can get a hair transplant, while people who have other types of hair loss, like bald patches, usually can't get one.

Personal care

Tips for healthy hair[138, 139]

How you wash your hair can make a big difference in how smooth and shiny it stays. Dermatologists have given you these easy tips to keep your hair healthy:

- How often you wash your hair should be based on how much oil your scalp produces. You might need to wash your hair more than once a day if it is oily. If you use chemicals on your hair, it might be drier, so you might want to wash it less often. Maybe you don't need to shampoo as often as you used to because your skin makes less oil as you age, on the other hand your hair might not be clean enough if it has flakes. This can lead to dandruff and other scalp diseases.

[138] American Academy of Dermatology - https://www.aad.org/public/everyday-care/hair-scalp-care/hair/healthy-hair-tips (Accessed in May 2024)

[139] American Academy of Dermatology - https://www.aad.org/public/everyday-care/hair-scalp-care/hair/habits-that-damage-hair (Accessed in May 2024)

- When you wash your hair, don't wash the whole length of hair; instead, focus on cleaning the scalp. If you only wash your hair, it can get dull, stiff, and fly away.
- If you don't use a "2-in-1" shampoo that cleans and conditions hair, use conditioner after every wash. Applying a conditioner can greatly enhance the look of worn-out or damaged hair by adding shine, lowering static electricity, making the hair stronger, and protecting it from UV rays. Put most of the conditioner on the hair's ends, and it shouldn't be used on the scalp or the length of the hair, because it can make fine hair look limp.
- Choose a shampoo and conditioner that are made for your hair type. For instance, if you dye your hair, you should use a shampoo made for dyed hair. A "2-in-1" shampoo might help if your hair is damaged or has been chemically treated. There are a lot of shampoo and conditioner brands that all do the same good things, regardless of the cost.
- Put a towel around your hair to soak up the water. Let your hair dry naturally, and don't rub it with a towel.
- Is your hair straight? Do not use a wide-tooth comb right away because your hair needs some time to dry. Do you have loose curls or hair that is wavy? Use a wide-tooth comb to comb your hair while it's damp. When your hair is wet, don't brush it.
- If you want to use a hair dryer, turn the heat down the least. Don't use a hot comb or curling iron on your hair for too long. Try to use these tools no more than once a week, or even less often.
- Keep your hair safe when you swim. Make sure chlorine doesn't damage your hair by washing and conditioning it before you go swimming. Wear a swim cap that fits snugly and use a shampoo and deep conditioner made just for swimmers to replace the moisture you lose while you swim.
- Wear your hair pulled back loosely or try a hairstyle that doesn't need styling tools that hold it for a long time. Covered rubber bands made just for styling hair should be used. There are other

ways to style your hair that won't pull it back too much, like a ponytail, bun, or cornrows.

- Only wear weaves and extensions when they are not heavy, so they don't pull. A salon that deals in weaves and hair extensions is the best place to get them. After getting a weave or hair extension, don't wear it for more than 2 or 3 months, and change up your haircuts every so often so you don't have to wear them all the time. When you wear a weave or hair extension, make sure you keep your scalp clean.
- Try to wait longer between touch-ups if you dye, smooth, or perm your hair, especially when the hair is dry. Try to wait at least 8 to 10 weeks between touch-ups in the winter. You should only get one service, like a perm, relaxer, or coloring, but if you want more than one service, perm or relax your hair first, and do it 2 weeks before you color your hair. Wear a wide-brimmed hat or use a leave-in conditioner with zinc oxide to protect your hair from the sun.
- Comb and brush your hair only to style it, you don't need to brush your hair 100 times a day. Moreover, when you comb your hair, be gentle and use a wide-tooth comb, don't pull and tug on it. Carefully get rid of knots and if needed, use a moisturizing conditioner.

How often should you shower?[140]

There is **no perfect number** of times to shower, but most people only need to do it a few times a week, unless they are dirty, sweaty, or have another reason to do it more often. It might be enough to take short showers of 3 or 4 minutes, and to focus on the armpits and groin.

Normal, healthy skin keeps a layer of oil on top of it and the right amount of "good" **bacteria** and other germs. These come off when you

---

[140] Harvard Health Publishing - https://www.health.harvard.edu/blog/showering-daily-is-it-necessary-2019062617193 (Published in August 2021)

wash and scrub, especially when the water is hot, so if you take a shower or bath every day, your skin might get dry, sensitive, or itchy. If your skin is dry and cracked, bacteria and allergens may be able to get through the barrier that skin is meant to provide, and this can lead to skin infections and allergic reactions. Normal germs can be killed by antibacterial soaps, but this throws off the balance of microorganisms on the skin and makes it easier for tougher organisms that are better at fighting off antibiotics. Normal microorganisms, dirt, and other things in our surroundings need to stimulate our immune systems in a certain way so that they can make protective antibodies and **"immune memory".** This is one reason why some doctors and dermatologists say kids shouldn't take baths every day. Taking a lot of baths or showers over a lifetime may make the immune system less effective.
You might also not want to take your daily shower because the water we use to clean ourselves may have salts, heavy metals, chlorine, fluoride, herbicides, and other chemicals in it, and it's possible that these will also cause trouble.

Then, the oils, perfumes, and other things that are added to shampoos, conditioners, and soaps may also cause problems, like **allergic reactions**, and they also **cost** a lot.
Finally, baths and showers **waste** a lot of **water**.

Cleaning ears

Putting something in your ear is not a good idea, according to doctors. Your ears **clean themselves** most of the time, so you don't need to do anything extra.
You should only clean them to get rid of or smooth the **earwax** that's on the outside of your ears.[141]
Earwax can't be stopped, and it keeps dirt and germs out of your ears.

---

[141] WebMD - https://www.webmd.com/skin-problems-and-treatments/how-to-clean-your-ear (Reviewed in September 2023)

However, hearing loss, earaches, the feeling that your ears are blocked, ringing, or buzzing in your ears (tinnitus), and vertigo are all **signs** of too much earwax deposits.

To **get rid** of this excess of earwax, don't use your fingers or anything else, like cotton buds. It will get worse pushing it in.
It's normal for earwax to come out on its own, but if it doesn't work and your ear gets clogged, put 2 to 3 drops of medical-grade almond or olive oil in it 3 to 4 times a day, for 3 to 5 days. Put your head on one side and use a dropper to put oil in your ear and wait a few minutes to let the oil work. Getting this done first thing in the morning and then right before bed may help you.
Also talk to a doctor or pharmacist about removing earwax in your ears, since they can offer help and treatment ideas. After about a week, the earwax should either fall out on its own or break down.[142]

Oral hygiene[143]

To lower your chance of caries and gum disease, it's important to do the right oral care at home for the right amount of time.
Some **general tips** on how to avoid cavities and gingivitis:

- Brush your teeth
- Floss - Clean between your teeth
- Eat a healthy diet that limits sugary drinks and snacks
- See your dentist regularly: tailor your recall interval to individual need based on assessed risk of disease

---

[142] National Health Service - https://www.nhs.uk/conditions/earwax-build-up (Reviewed in January 2024)
[143] American Dental Association - https://www.ada.org/en/resources/research/science-and-research-institute/oral-health-topics/home-care (Published in December 2022)

Brush your teeth correctly[144]

Brush your teeth **twice a day** with a fluoride toothpaste[145]

1. Hold your toothbrush at a 45 degrees angle to your gums.
2. Move the brush back and forth slowly in short, tooth-wide strokes.
3. Clean the outside, inside, and chewing areas of your teeth.
4. Tilt the toothbrush vertically and make several up-and-down strokes to clean the inside of the front teeth.
5. Brush your teeth for 2 minutes, which is 4 seconds per tooth.
6. Spit out any extra toothpaste after you brush your teeth. Don't rinse your mouth immediately after brushing, as it'll wash away the concentrated fluoride in the remaining toothpaste. It loses some of its antibacterial properties when you rinse it off.

Watch this video to see an animation prepared by National Health Service on how to brush your teeth correctly:
https://youtu.be/BapR9J86ZZw?si=oABzbVDZp46lyAmk

[144] National Health Service - https://www.nhs.uk/live-well/healthy-teeth-and-gums/how-to-keep-your-teeth-clean/ (Published in February 2022)
[145] American Dental Association - https://www.mouthhealthy.org/all-topics-a-z/brushing-your-teeth (Accessed in May 2024)

While this video prepared by Oral B, shows the right process in case you use an electric brush:
https://youtu.be/UUXAivWbnOw?si=_9aAPntu8Lnu6kRQ

A **toothbrush** with a small head and a tight, angled set of long and short round-end bristles works well for most people. Also, most people do best with bristles that are medium to soft. Whether you use an electric or hand toothbrush doesn't matter: they are both good as long as you use fluoride toothpaste and clean all the sides of your teeth, but some people like using an electric toothbrush because it helps them clean their teeth better. Every 3 to 4 months, or sooner if the bristles are worn, you should get a new toothbrush, because if your toothbrush is worn out, it won't clean your teeth well.

It's important to use **toothpaste** that has the right amount of **fluoride**. Find out how much fluorine each brand has by looking at the package:

- Toothpaste for adults should have at least 1,350 parts per million (ppm) of fluoride in it. Depending on your needs, your doctor may tell you to use toothpaste with more fluoride.
- Kids don't need to use toothpaste made just for them. No matter what age, kids can use family toothpaste as long as it has 1,350 to 1,500ppm of fluoride.
- Don't let kids lick or eat toothpaste from the tube.

When looking for toothpaste, think about what you need. Many people, especially those who brush their teeth well, don't need anything else besides fluoride to keep their teeth healthy. If you are worried about things like sensitivity, enamel wear, or whiter teeth, it is important to know what a toothpaste promises and whether the evidence backs them up:[146]

- **Sensitivity**: Any toothpaste that helps lower sensitivity will work better if you cut down on acidic foods and drinks between meals. Your hypersensitivity might go away on its own over time, or it might only happen sometimes. You should always see a doctor to make sure there aren't any other problems going on.
- **Whitening**: So as long as you don't have expectations that a whitening toothpaste will change the underlying color of your tooth enamel, there may be value in buying a toothpaste which makes whitening claims, because it might have ingredients that get rid of stains that a regular paste won't have.
- **Enamel wear**: There have been some improvements in this area in the last few years, and there may be good reasons to choose a toothpaste that is made to fix enamel, but keep in mind that all toothpastes with fluoride protect against enamel loss in some way. Also, many enamel repair claims are based on fluoride, which hardens or "remineralizes" enamel, so you don't have to spend a lot of money on toothpaste because even cheap ones have this in them.

Tooth decay can be avoided by using a **mouthwash** with fluoride. But don't use any mouthwash, even one with fluoride, right after brushing your teeth, because it will wash away the concentrated fluoride that was left on your teeth by the toothpaste. If you want to use mouthwash, pick a different time, like after lunch. After you use a fluoride rinse, don't eat or drink for 30 minutes.

[146] Which? - https://www.which.co.uk/reviews/electric-toothbrushes/article/choosing-the-best-toothpaste-a5QlY0j8jkeT (Published June 2023)

Flossing[147]

"Flossing" is a popular, shorthand word for cleaning the **space between your teeth** every day. There might not be a single "best" way to clean between teeth, like dental floss, interdental brushes, mouth irrigators, or wood sticks. Instead, the best way for each patient will be the one they use most often. Before you brush your teeth, it's the best moment to floss.

1. Grab 30 to 45 cm of dental floss or tape so that you have 3 to 4 cm of it taut between your hands.
2. Put as much dental floss or tape as you can between your teeth and into the space between your teeth and gums.
3. Do 8–10 sweeps of the floss up and down between each tooth to get rid of food and plaque.

If there are spaces between your teeth, you don't have to floss, instead, you can use interdental brushes or single-tufted brushes. The brush should fit between your teeth very well. To get rid of food stuck between your teeth, never use a stick, since you could hurt your gums, which could cause an infection.

Watch this video of the American Dental Association on how to floss your teeth correctly:
https://youtu.be/HhdoPXNKNm4?si=CDkOdDQzS4qa26Lf

[147] National Health Service - https://www.nhs.uk/live-well/healthy-teeth-and-gums/how-to-keep-your-teeth-clean (Published in February 2022)

How To Maintain White Teeth[148]

It doesn't matter if your teeth are already white or if you just finished a whitening treatment, you still need to do some work to keep that beautiful smile. If you want your teeth to stay white, you should be careful about how you treat them, just like you wouldn't drive through mud puddles after washing your car.

Here are some **tips** that will help your teeth stay whiter for longer:

- Keep **staining liquids** to a minimum: if you drink a coffee every morning and a cola every afternoon, you might notice that your teeth aren't as white as they used to be. Many drinks, like coffee, tea, cola, and red wine, can stain your teeth. If you really want to keep your teeth white, try drinking less of these things. If you can't live without these drinks, try drinking them through a straw, because when you drink through a straw, your teeth don't come into touch with as much liquid. You can even buy a set of straws that you can use more than once.
- **Drink water** between drinks that might stain: aside from being good for your health, water can also help get rid of dark liquids that stick to your teeth. Switch between a sip of water and a sip of coffee, tea, or hot chocolate.
- **Clean your teeth** after: more staining will happen if the drink stays on your teeth for a longer time. Bring toothpaste and a toothbrush with you so you can clean up after your coffee break. If you drink something acidic, like coffee, you must wait at least 30 minutes before brushing your teeth. You might spread the acid around your teeth instead of getting rid of it if you brush too soon.
- Get rid of **tobacco**: quitting tobacco is good for more than just keeping your teeth white. When you smoke, you put your mouth at risk for many problems, such as gum disease, oral

[148] Colgate - https://www.colgate.com/en-us/oral-health/teeth-whitening/how-to-maintain-white-teeth (Updated in March 2023)

cancer, loss of taste, and slower healing after some dental treatments. Quitting smoking can make a huge difference in how your teeth look and your general dental health.

- Make sure you **take care** of your teeth every day: Since plaque attracts staining substances, reducing plaque, in general, will reduce overall discoloration.
- **Get your teeth cleaned** regularly by your dentist: when your doctor or dental hygienist cleans your teeth, they can polish away surface stains. The rough surface of a professional cleaning can help fight discoloration without having to bleach your teeth again.

More and more people are spending money to make their teeth whiter and better. Whitening involves bleaching your teeth to make them lighter. It won't make your teeth completely white, but it will make the color a few shades lighter. Tooth whitening can be done by any dentist, while there are risks with home kits. Whiter teeth don't last forever: they can last anywhere from a few months to 3 years, depending on the person. No matter what you do, the chemicals used in teeth whitening could make your gums sensitive, and especially if you already have sensitive teeth.[149]

Chewing gums[150]

Different kinds of chewing gum have been around for a very **long time**. Anthropology and dentistry have come together at an archeological site in Sweden to find lumps of birch bark tar with tooth impressions of children and teens from 9,000 years ago. This is the oldest proof that people chewed on substances that look like gum. A related substance, called mastic, was chewed on by the ancient Greeks, so the word "mastication" likely comes from this word. Native Americans and the

---

[149] National Health Service - https://www.nhs.uk/conditions/teeth-whitening (Reviewed in January 2022)

[150] American Dental Association - https://www.ada.org/en/resources/research/science-and-research-institute/oral-health-topics/chewing-gum (Updated in May 2023)

Inuit used to chew gum from spruce trees, and Europeans who came to New England picked up this habit.

Chewing gum makes your **saliva** flow and amount increases by stimulating taste receptors in your mouth and working mechanically.
Getting more saliva to flow may help protect against tooth cavities in a number of ways. More saliva means more calcium and phosphate ions, which can help remineralize tooth enamel. The fluoride in the saliva can replace the enamel's magnesium and carbonate with fluorapatite crystals, which are harder and less likely to break down. Acids in foods or drinks can soften the enamel on your teeth, but saliva can protect them. Swallowing extra saliva made by stimulation also gets rid of acid, since if you don't trigger your saliva, it doesn't have much of a buffering effect against acid, having more protein, sodium, calcium, chloride, and bicarbonate. Saliva also adds proteins to the sides of teeth, making an acquired enamel pellicle that keeps teeth from wearing down.
If you regularly brush your teeth twice a day with fluoridated toothpaste and clean between your teeth every day, chewing sugar-free gum may still help lower your chance of cavities.

If you grind your teeth at night (**bruxism**), don't chew gum. It makes your jaw muscles more used to clenching, which will make you more likely to do it again.[151]

Bad breath[152]

A lot of people have bad breath, called **halitosis**, you may treat it yourself:

- At least twice a day, brush your teeth and gums gently for 2 minutes.
- Use fluoride toothpaste.

---

[151] WebMD - https://www.webmd.com/oral-health/teeth-grinding-bruxism (Reviewed in December 2023)

[152] National Health Service - https://www.nhs.uk/conditions/bad-breath (Reviewed in December 2021)

- Clean your tongue gently once a day with a tongue scraper or cleaner.
- At least once a day, clean between your teeth with interdental brushes or floss.
- Get regular dental check-ups.
- Keep your dentures clean and take them out at night.
- After eating or drinking something strong-smelling, chew sugar-free mint or gum.
- Try antibacterial mouthwash or toothpaste.

Excessive sweating[153]

The body's sweat glands release water when you sweat, and this helps your body to **stay cool**.
How much you sweat is based on how many sweat **glands** you have, and the sweat glands in men work more often.
About 2 to 4 million sweat glands are present in each person at birth, and they start to work fully when a person hits puberty.

The **autonomic nerve system** is in charge of sweating.
Things that can make you sweat more are being in hot weather, working out, or being in situations that make you scared, nervous, angry, or ashamed. Some foods, like those with monosodium glutamate, caffeine (chocolate, coffee, tea), hot sauce, spices like curry or cumin, and booze can also be triggers.
After sweating a lot, you should drink a lot of water or electrolyte-containing drinks like sports drinks to replace the sweat you lost. You should also cool down a bit to stop sweating even more, and if the salt from your sweat has dried on your skin, wash your face and body.
Both not sweating enough and sweating too much can be bad. Not sweating can be dangerous because it makes you more likely to get too

---

[153] American Academy of Dermatology Association - https://www.aad.org/public/diseases/a-z/hyperhidrosis-self-care (Accessed in May 2024)

hot, and it's possible that excessive sweating is worse for your mental health than for your body.

A lot of people who sweat too much (**hyperhidrosis**) don't know that they have a medical condition that can be treated.
Get checked out by a dermatologist, because he or she will be able to tell you what kind of hyperhidrosis you have and suggest the best way to treat it.
It's important to use an **antiperspirant** instead of perfume, since antiperspirants can help you sweat less. They cover up or get rid of body odor, but they let you breathe. Before going to bed, put antiperspirant on dry skin.

Have **sweaty feet**? Take care of yourself by following these tips. You are more likely to get foot odor and skin infections like athlete's foot if your feet stay wet or cold. Dermatologists say:

- When you can, wear sandals
- Wear shoes made from leather that comes from nature. This lets air flow through
- Take your shoes off when you can
- Don't wear the same shoes twice in a row. Let the shoes dry all the way through before you put them on again
- Wear socks that keep your feet dry. Cotton socks don't get rid of sweat. It will say on the package if the socks can wick away sweat
- Change your socks every day, or more often if they get wet
- Clean your socks before using them again

Deodorant[154]

Antiperspirants and deodorants are now common parts of many people's daily hygiene habits.
You may have heard that some chemicals in deodorants and antiperspirants can cause **breast cancer** or problems with the **kidneys**. But is it true?
The National Kidney Foundation only warns people with very weak kidneys about the health risks of using antiperspirants, and the American Cancer Society found that claims that deodorants can cause breast cancer are not backed up by sound science.
The chemicals made from **aluminum** are used a lot in cosmetics and medicines, and aluminum salts are what keep you from sweating and are found in antiperspirants. The salts need to break down so that sweat doesn't build up on top of your pores. If you have kidney problems, especially if your kidneys only work about 30% of the time or less, aluminum might be a bigger problem for you. This is why the US Food and Drug Administration (FDA) makes antiperspirant makers put in labels just for people with kidney disease.

[154] Penn Medicine - https://www.pennmedicine.org/updates/blogs/health-and-wellness/2019/june/deodorant (Published in June 2019)

The world of disabilities

"Once we accept our limits, we can surpass them".
Albert Einstein (theoretical physicist)

People are living longer, but they have more health problems. A lot of the time, the illnesses and diseases that kill the most people also take away the most good life-years. About 16% of the world's population, or **1.3 billion people**, have a major disability today.

The World Health Organization says that disability has **3 parts**:

- A problem with the way a person's body works or looks, or with how their mind works. Loss of a limb, loss of vision, or memory loss are all examples of disabilities

- Limitations on activities, like not being able to see or hear well, walk, or solve problems
- There are limits on normal daily activities like working, going to social and leisure events, and getting medical care and preventive services

Senses[155]

What number of senses does a person have? There are many answers to this question, since it's not agreed upon whether we have **7, 9, 10, or 12 senses**. Which answer is right? It relies on how you explain things.

First, we should note that all of the numbers in the last sentence are **bigger than 5**. It doesn't take much thought to realize that people have more than the 5 "classical" senses: **hearing, vision, taste, smell, and touch**.
The idea of 5 ancient senses goes back at least to Aristotle. He says that there is a sense organ for every sense in De Anima (Of the Soul).

The eyes, ears, nose, tongue, skin, and vestibular system are the 6 sense organs you count.
The **vestibular system** has been known to work as a sense organ since the early 1800s, which is more than 2,000 years after Aristotle. Now, we understand that the vestibular system in the inner ear is a key part of how we keep our balance. It's also very important for vision, as it lets us keep both eyes on something even when our heads move.

Let's make a few changes to Aristotle's explanation of what a sense is. If you don't have a sense organ, you just need a different kind of sensitive receptor for each sense. There are at least 4 types of sensory sensors in the skin alone. These are for touch, **temperature**, **pain**, and **proprioception**, which means knowing where your body is in space. A sensory receptor is a special kind of cell that gets electrical messages

[155] John Hopkins - https://www.press.jhu.edu/newsroom/how-many-senses-do-we-have (Published in February 2012)

from certain kinds of stimuli and sends them to the brain. Rods and cones in the eye are nerve cells that pick up on sensations, and when light of different wavelengths and intensities hits them, they send messages. There are so many sensitive receptors in the skin that they are optimized for more than just touch. Different temperature sensors are best for different temperature ranges, and there are at least 6 types of them.

Healthy vision

First, a few **curiosities** about our eyes.
Your eyes are an extension of your brain and are wired straight to it.
The orbicularis oculi are the body's fastest-moving muscle; it can contract in less than 1/100th of a second. A blink lasts between 100 and 150 milliseconds most of the time. Did you know that when you talk, you blink more than when you read? That's why reading makes you tired.
People with blue eyes have only been around for 6,000 to 10,000 years, and before that, everyone had brown eyes, so if you have blue eyes it's because you had a relative who lived around the Black Sea. People with green eyes make up only 2% of the population, and most of them live in Ireland, Scotland, and Northern Europe. Babies' eyes are either blue or brown when they are born, and getting green eyes can take anywhere from 6 months to 3 years.
It's not true that eyes stay the same size from birth, but a baby's eyes are about 75% the size of an adult eye.

Around the world, 285 million people have trouble seeing, and 39 million of them are blind. However, 80% of vision loss can be avoided or fixed.[156]

[156] Novartis - https://www.novartis.com/stories/eye-fastest-muscle-human-body (Published in June 2016)

Taking care of your eyes starts with you, so follow these ideas:[157]

- Watch what you **eat** to keep your eyes healthy, since a well-balanced diet will help your eyes stay healthy. Getting lots of different kinds of fruits and vegetables is important. Leafy greens like spinach, kale, and collard greens are wonderful. It has been shown that fish like salmon, tuna, and halibut are good for your eyes as well.
- Get **moving**. If you are overweight or obese, you may be more likely to get diabetes and other diseases that can make it hard to see.
- Say something if your view **changes**. Do you have fuzzy vision? Do you often squint? Do you ever have trouble seeing? Talk to your doctor whether your eyes hurt or if you notice any changes in how you see.
- Stay away from **germs**. You should always wash your hands before putting them near your eyes, especially when you're putting in or taking out contacts.
- **Gear up**. To keep your eyes safe, wear the right gear. Better safety habits, like wearing safety glasses, can help keep your eyes from getting hurt.
- Keep cool and put on your **shades**. The sun can make your eyes hurt. The best sunglasses will stop 100% of both UVA and UVB sun rays. Also, remember not to look at the sun straight on.
- Take a **break** for your eyes. A lot of the time, do you stare at your phone, computer, or TV? If you look at one thing for too long, it can hurt your eyes. The 20-20-20 rule says to look 20 feet (6 meters) away for 20 seconds every 20 minutes to give your eyes a break.
- Say no to **smoking**. If you smoke, you might get some pretty bad eye problems that could eventually blind you.

---

[157] National Eye Institute - https://www.nei.nih.gov/learn-about-eye-health/nei-for-kids/healthy-vision-tips (Updated in August 2023)

Vision problems like amblyopia, strabismus, and major refractive errors are the most common conditions that make it hard for kids in the United States. It is more likely that treatment will work if it is found early, but less than 15% of preschoolers get an eye check and less than 22% of preschoolers get some kind of vision screening. Eye exams for kids got the same score as exams for women to check for breast cancer.
Vision problems in people younger than 40 are mostly caused by refractive mistakes (which affect 25% of kids and teens) and eye injuries that happen by accident. Every year, about one million eye injuries happen, and 90% of them could have been avoided. Over half of all people who get eye injuries are between the ages of 18 and 45.
People ages 40 and up are most likely to get cataracts, diabetic retinopathy, glaucoma, and age-related macular degeneration. In their early stages, these diseases often don't show any symptoms. The number of people who are blind or have trouble seeing rises quickly with age, especially after age 75.[158]

Hearing[159]

It is expected that by 2050, almost 2.5 billion people will have some degree of **hearing loss**, and at least 700 million of them will need to get help to improve their hearing. Over 1 billion young people are at risk of permanent hearing loss that can be avoided because they listen in ways that are not safe.
More than 5% of the world's people, or 430 million people, need therapy for their hearing loss.

Hearing loss of more than 35 **decibels** (dB) in the better ear is called "**disabling**". Nearly 80% of people who can't hear well live in low- or middle-income countries. Hearing loss is more common as people get

---

[158] Centers for Disease Control and Prevention - https://www.cdc.gov/visionhealth/risk/age.htm (Reviewed in December 2022)
[159] World Health Organization - https://www.who.int/news-room/fact-sheets/detail/deafness-and-hearing-loss (Published in February 2023)

older, and more than 25% of people older than 60 have hearing loss that makes it hard for them to do things.

Causes of hearing loss are:[160]

- One of the main reasons is **loud noise**. The inner ear can be hurt by noise from lawn mowers, snow blowers, or loud music, which can lead to lasting hearing loss. If you turn down the sound on your devices, move away from loud noise, or use earplugs or other ear protection, you can avoid most hearing loss caused by noise.
  Decibels are the numbers used to measure sound. Even if they are heard for a long time, sounds at or below 70 A-weighted decibels (dBA) probably won't damage your hearing. But being exposed to sounds at or above 85 dBA for a long time or over and over again can damage your hearing. There is less time for noise-induced hearing loss to happen when the sound is louder. Here are the average decibel levels of some well-known sounds: most conversations (60–70 dBA), movies (74–104 dBA), motorcycles and dirt bikes (80–110 dBA), concerts, sports events, and music played through headphones at full volume (94–110 dBA), sirens (110–129 dBA), and fireworks shows (140–160 dBA).
  The 2021 study found that people who wear headphones in a place that is already noisy are 4.5 times more likely to lose their hearing. The 60/60 rule says that you should only use your MP3 player at up to 60% of its highest volume for a total of 60 minutes a day
- **Earwax** or fluid buildup can reduce your hearing by blocking sounds that are sent from the eardrum to the inner ear. If wax buildup is a problem, your doctor may suggest gentle ways to get rid of it. Look at the exact part of this book that talks about earwax

[160] National Institute of Aging - https://www.nia.nih.gov/health/hearing-loss-common-problem-older-adults (Reviewed in January 2023)

- **Torn eardrum**. Infections, pressure, or putting things in the ear, like cotton-tipped swabs, can hurt the eardrum. If you have pain in your ears or fluid draining from one of them, you should see a doctor
- **Diabetes and high blood pressure**. A heart problem, stroke, brain injury, or a tumor may also make it hard for you to hear. So can ear infections from viruses and bacteria (also called otitis media)
- Taking some **medicines** that hurt the inner ear, sometimes permanently. People who have serious infections, cancer, or heart problems may take these medicines. Some medicines and even aspirin in some doses are included as well. Talk to your doctor if you have any problems while taking a medicine
- Differences in **genes**. Not all types of hearing loss that are passed down are noticeable at birth, and some forms can change over time. As an example, otosclerosis is thought to be a disease that is passed down through families, and it is marked by abnormal bone growth that makes it hard for parts inside the ear to work properly

When you **talk to someone who has trouble hearing**, here are some things you can do:

- When you talk to a group of people, make sure that people who have trouble hearing are included.
- Talk in a quiet place to block out background noise, especially in restaurants and social events.
- Stand where there is good lighting and use your body language or facial emotions to give hints.
- Face the person and be clear when you talk. Maintain eye contact.
- You can speak a little louder, but don't yell.
- Speak slowly and easily as much as possible.
- Don't cover your mouth, eat, or chew gum while you talk.
- If you have to, say it again, but this time use different words.
- Try to let one person talk at a time.

- Be patient. Some people who have hearing loss may also be angry about it. Stay calm and upbeat.
- Ask what you can do to help.

Mobility issues[161]

Age makes a lot of people worry that they will not be able to move around as well. They're afraid they won't be able to do the things they love, go to the places they love, or even do the things they need to do every day.

Being able to move around freely and easily is called mobility. It's important for working well and living on your own. As we age, our ability to move around may change, and these changes happen for many reasons, such as changes in our balance, strength, and gait (how we walk).

All of these things can make it harder for older people to do their own things and go out to see friends and family, moreover they can make falls more likely and more serious.

Risks factors for mobility issues are:

- When older people are **hospitalized, fall, or have a movement problem** like Parkinson's disease, they often lose the ability to do certain things physically.
- Not getting **enough exercise** can also make it more likely that someone will lose their mobility as they age.
- The rising number of people who are **sedentary** (sitting too much) is a growing health worry. There are too many older people who don't move around enough and who sit for too long every day, about 9 to 13 hours on average. Scientists are looking into this problem and trying to build up enough scientific evidence to help make public health recommendations on how

[161] National Institute of Aging - https://www.nia.nih.gov/news/maintaining-mobility-and-preventing-disability-are-key-living-independently-we-age (Published in November 2020)

to break people's habits of being sedentary in ways that support healthy aging.

Back pain[162, 163]

Low Back Pain (LBP) affected 619 million people around the world in 2020. The number of cases is expected to rise to 843 million by 2050, mostly because people are living longer and increasing in number.
Low back pain (LBP) is the **most common cause of disability** in the world and the condition for which the most people can benefit from therapy. Anyone of any age can get LBP, and most people will experience it at least once in their life.
Up to age 80, the frequency goes up, but the most cases of LBP happen in people aged 50 to 55, and women are more likely than men to have them.
It's called **non-specific** LBP when the pain can't be linked to a specific disease or structural reason. This is the case in about 90% of cases.

Self-care is a key part of dealing with LBP and getting back to doing things that are important to you.
Rehabilitation is important for all types and stages of LBP because it helps people feel better, understand their pain, come up with ways to speed up their healing, and make their lives better.
To ease the pain and stop future episodes of non-specific low back pain, you can stay active and try to keep up with your daily activities, do some back pain exercises and stretches, improve your mental health, keep your weight in a healthy range, stop smoking, get enough sleep, stay involved in work and social activities, make changes to your workspace that are better for your body, and don't stay in bed for long time.

---

[162] World Health Organization - https://www.who.int/news-room/fact-sheets/detail/low-back-pain (Published in June 2023)
[163] John Hopkins - https://www.hopkinsmedicine.org/health/conditions-and-diseases/back-pain/addressing-neck-and-back-pain-when-youre-working-from-home (Accessed in May 2024)

People don't think much about **sitting**, but bad balance while sitting can make back and neck pain worse. At first, sitting up straight might seem a little odd or even awkward, and this is because we're used to sitting in chairs that don't support us well or because we slouch when we're down. Bad posture and the way we sit can become habits that make us feel at ease.

The key to sitting right is keeping the natural "S" shape curves in your spine. This is a key part of getting rid of back pain. When you sit like this, your weight and gravity are spread out properly, so your muscles don't have to work hard to keep you in an odd position. While we don't expect you to always sit up straight, try to make this one of the things you do while sitting down.

People with back pain want to be able to sit for longer periods of time and in comfort. Instead of sitting for long amounts of time, we should get up and move around.

Try to stand up every 30 minutes, even if it's just to stretch and move around. A lot of people work with their heads forward while they're on video meetings or working on paper.

Some ways to spend less time sitting down:[164]

- Try to take **breaks** from screens every so often. For example, if you're watching TV, get up every time there is an ad. Take breaks from your computer screen every so often at work, get some water, go for a walk around the block, or talk to a coworker. Setting a reminder on your phone or putting a post-it note on your screen at eye level can help you remember to take breaks.
- When you can, **stand up** instead of sitting down. Do it for small amounts of time while you watch TV, are in a meeting, are at your desk, or are on the phone. Standing desks are also being used in offices by more and more businesses. According to a study, these desks might help workers feel less tired and be

[164] British Heart Foundation - https://www.bhf.org.uk/informationsupport/heart-matters-magazine/activity/sitting-down/spend-less-time-sitting-down (Accessed in May 2024)

more productive. If you think this would help you, you might want to talk to your HR department. As you stand at the desk, it's fine to move your weight from one foot to the other. The catch is that we need to use our muscles, especially our hips, when we do this. We rely too much on passive tissues to support us during the day instead of using our muscles to stand up straight against gravity.

- Plan to be **active** at times when you normally don't do much. For example, instead of heating up a ready-made meal in the evening, you could go to an exercise class, go for a walk, or cook a healthy meal from scratch. You could even get some exercise on your way to work by walking part of the way before getting on the bus or for a ride to home.
- Limit your **time** spent doing things that don't involve moving. For example, you could only watch TV for an hour in the evening or not read emails or use the internet during certain times of the day. It's good for everyone in the family to follow these rules.

While a bed, armchair, or sofa is great for resting, it might not be the best place to work for hours on end.

If you spend a lot of time in front of a screen, having the right **ergonomics** and a **good chair** can help your balance and keep your back from getting sore.

Arm rests that move forward and back are what you need, not just up and down. As you sit in the chair, your arms should be about 90 degrees apart so that you don't have to reach.

Support for your lumbar spine is important. You should be able to move the chair so that it fits your lower back, and it should be high enough for your feet to touch the floor. You can get your legs to reach the floor by putting something under your feet.

The middle row of keys on the computer should be level with your forearm and elbow, and your arms should be parallel to the floor. Desk feet can be used to raise the desk if it's not at the right height. Use a foot stool to raise the seat height if it's too high. Put the mouse close to the keyboard so it's easy to get to.

Place the screen in front of the person at eye level and at arm's length.

If you use your phone for work more than 40% of the time, you might want to get a hands-free set.

Healthy lifestyles

"Your genetics load the gun. Your lifestyle pulls the trigger"
Mehmet Oz (television presenter and physician)

Eating healthy

What we eat makes us who we are.

Eating healthy keeps you from getting heart disease, diabetes, cancer, and many other chronic noncommunicable diseases.

Based on what the WHO says, here is some helpful **information** about how to eat well and the benefits of doing so:[165]

---

[165] World Health Organization - https://www.who.int/initiatives/behealthy/healthy-diet (Accessed in May 2024)

- Feed babies and young kids **breast milk**.
  A healthy diet starts early in life. Breastfeeding helps babies grow and develop normally, and it may also have health benefits in the long run, like lowering the chance of becoming overweight or obese and getting noncommunicable diseases. From birth to 6 months, kids should only be fed breast milk. Also, starting to give your baby a variety of safe and healthy extra foods at 6 months is important, and you should still nurse your child until at least 2 years old.
- Get a lot of **fruits and veggies**.
  A lot of vitamins, minerals, fiber, plant protein, and antioxidants can be found in them. If you cook fruits and veggies for too long, you may lose some important vitamins. When you use canned or dried fruits and veggies, pick ones that don't have extra sugars or salt added to them. People who eat a lot of fruits and veggies are much less likely to be overweight, get heart disease, stroke, diabetes, and some types of cancer.
- Cut back on **fat**.
  There is a lot of energy in fats and oils, however heart disease and stroke risk go up when you eat too much, especially the wrong kinds of fat, like saturated fat and trans-fat made in factories. Instead of animal fats or oils high in saturated fats like butter, ghee, lard, coconut, and palm oil, use unsaturated veggie oils like olive, soy, sunflower, or corn oil. People shouldn't eat more than 30% of their daily calories from fat if they don't want to gain weight and limit saturated fat to less than 10% of calories a day. Instead of red meat, choose white meat (like chicken) and fish, which are usually low in fat. Processed foods are high in fat and salt, so don't eat too much of them. Also, try to choose milk and dairy items that are low in fat or have less fat.
- Cut down on **sugary** foods.
  Less than 10% of your total energy should come from sweets if you want to eat healthily. Getting it down to less than 5% is even better for your health. Picking fresh veggies over sweet snacks like cookies, cakes, and chocolate can help you eat less sugar.

Cutting back on pop, fruit juices, cordials, syrups, flavored milks, and yogurt drinks, which are all high in sugar, is another way to lower your sugar intake.

- Cut down on **salt**.
  A daily salt intake of less than 5 grams, or just under a teaspoon, can help avoid high blood pressure and lower the risk of heart disease and stroke in adults. Cutting back on salt and condiments high in salt, like soy sauce and fish sauce, when making and preparing food can help lower salt intake.

Obesity

Being overweight or obese means having an abnormally high amount of fat that is harmful to your health. We use your height and weight to find out if your weight is good. This is called the **Body Mass Index (BMI)**. To find an adult's BMI, split their weight in kilograms (kg) by the square of their height in meters (m). If you want to be healthy, your BMI should be between 18.5 and 24.9. If your BMI is over 25, you are overweight, and if it is over 30, you are obese. However, take into consideration that muscle mass weighs more than fat, but it's not taken into account in the BMI measurement.

The problem of obesity has become an **epidemic**. The global burden of disease report for 2017 says that being overweight or obese killed over 4 million people each year, and the number of overweight and obese children and adults is still rising. The number of overweight or obese kids and teens aged 5 to 19 around the world rose from 4% in 1975 to 18% by 2016. Currently 74% of people in the US are overweight or obese.[166] These days, there are more overweight than underweight people everywhere except sub-Saharan Africa and Asia. People used to think that overweight and obesity were only problems in high-income

---

[166] Dietary Guidelines for Americans - https://www.dietaryguidelines.gov/sites/default/files/2021-03/Dietary_Guidelines_for_Americans-2020-2025.pdf (Published in December 2020)

countries, but now they are becoming much more common in low- and middle-income countries, especially in cities. Most kids who are overweight or fat live in developing countries, where the rate of growth has been more than 30% higher than in developed countries.

Many of the things that lead to overweight and obesity can be **stopped or reversed**.[167]

You don't need to do everything at once, but just try one thing at a time until you find what works:[168]

- Get 150 minutes of **exercise** a week; you can do this in several shorter sessions.
- Aim to get 5 times a day 80 grams of fresh, canned, or frozen **fruit** or **veggies**.
- Don't go on a diet and lose weight **all at once**. Aim to lose 0.5 to 1 kg (1 to 2 pounds) per week.
- Read food **labels**.
- Drink **water** instead of sugary drinks. If you don't like the taste, add lemon, or lime slices.
- Cut back on foods that are high in **fat** and **sugar**. One way to start is to switch from sugary cereal to wholegrain cereal.
- Share your weight loss **plan** with someone you trust; they can keep you going when things go wrong.
- Don’t skip meals, you might eat more **snacks** because you're hungry.
- If your plate is already full, **don't eat everything** on it. You can save food for the next day.

---

[167] World Health Organization - https://www.who.int/health-topics/obesity (Accessed in May 2024)

[168] National Health Service - https://www.nhs.uk/live-well/healthy-weight/managing-your-weight/tips-to-help-you-lose-weight/ (Reviewed in March 2023)

To reduce carbs?

The only foods that don't have a lot of carbohydrates are dairy goods, which have milk sugar (lactose).
The body gets calories, or "energy," from carbohydrates, and there are 4 calories in every gram of carbs. Carbohydrates are broken down by the body into **glucose**, which is the main source of energy for the body's cells, tissues, and organs (like the brain and muscles). Glucose can be used right away or saved in the muscles and liver for later use.

Dietary **fiber** is a type of carbohydrate that is made up of many sugar molecules that are linked together in a way that makes it hard for the small intestine to break down. Fiber in the diet can help you go to the bathroom more often, lower your blood sugar and cholesterol, and lower the number of calories you eat. Dietary fiber includes the ones that come from plants, like nuts, peas, beans, fruits, veggies, seeds, and whole grains.

The **Daily Value (DV)** is 275 grams of total carbs every day, based on a regular diet of 2,000 calories. Your DV may be higher or lower than this, depending on how many calories you need.
Look at the %DV of total carbs when you are comparing and picking foods. Also, keep in mind that a serving with 5% DV or less of total carbs is low and a serving with 20% DV or more of total carbs is high.[169]

Some people can lower their total caloric intake by cutting back on or eliminating carbohydrates, but carbs are an **important** part of a healthy diet, so people shouldn't cut them out completely.
How many carbs you should eat varies on your age, weight, level of activity, and medical history, among other things. If you don't change anything else about your diet, cutting carbs might not help you lose

[169] Food and Drug Administration - https://www.accessdata.fda.gov/scripts/interactivenutritionfactslabel/assets/InteractiveNFL_TotalCarbohydrate_October2021.pdf (Published in October 2021)

weight as much as it could, and you might not get all the nutrients you need either.[170]

Low carb diets can help people lose weight more easily than other diets, as long as they stick to them. They can make people feel less hungry, which makes them eat fewer calories.[171]
However, a different study that looked only at obese people didn't find a big difference in weight loss 24 months after starting either a low-carbohydrate or low-fat diet.[172]
They show that a low-carb diet might help some people lose weight but might not be right for others.
Researchers have found that people lose an average of 13 pounds (6 kilograms) in a year. But the study also found that a low-fat diet can help people lose the same amount of weight in a year.[173]
Another study found that people who followed a low-carbohydrate diet for 8 weeks lost 22.8% of the visceral fat (also called "belly fat") in their bodies, while people who followed a low-fat diet only dropped 1%. The most dangerous kind of fat is visceral fat, which is highly linked to many diseases.[174]
A **big drop** in carbs all of a sudden can lead to short-term problems like nausea, headaches, and muscle cramps.

---

[170] Centers for Disease Control and Prevention - https://www.cdc.gov/diabetes/managing/eat-well/diabetes-and-carbohydrates.html (Reviewed in April 2023)
[171] Nutrition, Metabolism and Cardiovascular Diseases - https://www.ncbi.nlm.nih.gov/pmc/articles/PMC4873405/ (Published in June 2016)
[172] Frontiers in Nutrition - https://www.ncbi.nlm.nih.gov/pmc/articles/PMC9397119/ (Published in August 2022)
[173] Healthcare (Basel) – https://www.ncbi.nlm.nih.gov/pmc/articles/PMC6163457/ (Published in June 2018)
[174] Nutrition & Metabolism – https://nutritionandmetabolism.biomedcentral.com/articles/10.1186/s12986-020-00481-9 (Published in 2020)

If you don't eat enough carbs, your body may turn fat into ketones for energy with a process called **ketosis,** and this may cause bad breath, headaches, tiredness, and weakness.
It's not clear what kind of long-term health risks a low-carb diet might have. If you cut back on carbs for a long time, you might not get enough of some minerals or vitamins and have stomach problems.[175]

You can cut carbs out of your diet without making it feel too strict in a number of easy ways.
Here are some **easy ways** to cut back on carbs.[176]

- Eat less **processed bread and grains**. Bread is often the first thing that comes to mind when people think of carbs. The bread we eat today, especially white bread, has a lot of refined flour, not much fiber, and easy carbs. But, as a study points out, these highly processed grains might be worse for you than carbs from foods like fruits and veggies. A lot of people find it hard to give up sweetened and processed grains and bread, but it may be very important for people who want to lose weight by cutting carbs.
- Look for **options to flours**. Nut flours, like those made from walnuts, almonds, and acorns, may be great for people on a low-carb diet. A lot of people on a low-carb diet also use coconut flour instead. These low-carb flours can be used to make a lot of different foods. To fit them into their diet, people might try making fried chicken, pizza crusts, buns, and pancakes with them.
- As a side dish, try **whole grains** like brown rice, bulgur, couscous, and quinoa. Also, switch from refined to whole grain versions of foods you eat every day, like breads, cereals, pasta, and rice.

---

[175] Mayo Clinic - https://www.mayoclinic.org/healthy-lifestyle/weight-loss/in-depth/low-carb-diet/art-20045831 (Published in November 2022)
[176] Medical News Today - https://www.medicalnewstoday.com/articles/322988 (Updated in January 2024)

How many meals a day[177]

A lot of people still plan their days around "three square meals," but it may **not matter how many you eat**. If you want to lower your risk of heart disease and other health problems that come with being overweight, the most important thing is how you eat those meals.
Overall, a person's body size is still based on how many **calories** they eat. During the day, make sure you spread out the calories you eat, and also, don't skip meals.
Cutting out food might seem like a good way to lose weight, but it's not. Not giving your body food is bad for you, and because you're so hungry, you usually gain all those calories back plus some.

Intermittent fasting[178]

Intermittent fasting is an eating plan that switches between **fasting** and eating on a **regular schedule**. Research has shown that fasting every so often can help you control your weight and stop or even cure some diseases.
Our bodies have changed over time so that we can go for hours, days, or even longer without eating. In the past, before people learned how to farm, they were hunters and gatherers who learned how to go for long periods of time without eating and still do well. They had to because hunting animals and gathering nuts and berries took a lot of time and energy.
When you don't eat for hours, your body runs out of energy and starts burning fat instead (metabolic switching).

---

[177] American Heart Association - https://www.heart.org/en/healthy-living/healthy-eating/eat-smart/nutrition-basics/is-3-meals-a-day-the-only-way (Reviewed in December 2023)
[178] Johns Hopkins University - https://www.hopkinsmedicine.org/health/wellness-and-prevention/intermittent-fasting-what-is-it-and-how-does-it-work (Accessed in May 2024)

When you do intermittent fasting, you only eat at certain times. Intermittent fasting can be done in a number of **different ways**, but they all involve picking regular times to eat and not eat.

- The daily approach, which says you can only eat during 6- to 8-hour time every day. You could try 16/8 fasting, which means you eat for 8 hours and don't eat for 16.
- The 5:2 plan, which calls for eating normally 5 days a week. You can only eat one 500–600-calorie meal on the other 2 days. For example, let's say you decide to eat normally every day except Monday and Thursday. Those days would be your one-meal days.

Going without food for longer amounts of time, like 24–36–48–72 hours, may not be better for you and may even be dangerous. If you go too long without eating, your body might start storing more fat to make up for the lack of food.

It might take the body 2 to 4 weeks to get used to fasting. While you're getting used to the new schedule, you may feel hungry or irritable. Those who make it through the adjustment stage, on the other hand, are more likely to stick with the plan because they feel better.

During times when you're not eating, you can drink water and low-calorie drinks like black coffee and tea.

Keep in mind that going crazy during your eating times is not what "eating normally" means.

So far, study has shown the following **benefits** of intermittent fasting:

- Heart health. Intermittent fasting made measures of blood pressure, heart rate at rest, and other heart-related things better.
- Ability to think and remember.
- How well you do physically. Teenage guys who fasted for 16 hours lost fat but kept their muscle mass.
- Type 2 diabetes and being overweight
- Health of tissues. Animal studies showed that irregular fasting decreased tissue damage during surgery and led to better results.

Not everyone can do intermittent fasting. Your primary care doctor should know about any diet you want to try before you start intermittent fasting. It's not a good idea for kids and teens under 18 years old, women who are pregnant or breastfeeding, people with type 1 diabetes who take insulin, and people who have had eating disorders in the past.

Eat as a rainbow[179]

Every day, eating a range of fresh, unprocessed foods helps your body get the nutrients it needs. Also, staying away from foods that are high in sugar, fat, and salt is helpful. For young children's growth and development, eating healthy, **well-balanced** food is very important. Older people can live healthy and busier lives with it too.
There are many types of foods that the WHO says people should eat. These include cereals (like wheat, barley, rye, maize, or rice), starchy tubers or roots (like potato, yam, taro, or cassava), legumes (like lentils and beans), vegetables, fruit, and foods that come from animals (like meat, fish, eggs, and milk).

Mediterranean diet

The word "Mediterranean diet" refers to the traditional ways of eating in the countries that are close to the Mediterranean Sea. **There isn't just one** Mediterranean diet, because the Mediterranean is surrounded by at least 16 countries. There are differences in culture, ethnicity, religion, economy, geography, and agricultural production between these countries and even between areas within each country. These all affect how people eat.

There are, however, some **characteristics** that are the same:

- Lots of potatoes, beans, nuts, seeds, fruits, vegetables, and bread

---

[179] World Health Organization - https://www.who.int/news-room/questions-and-answers/item/healthy-diet-keys-to-eating-well (Published in October 2020)

- Olive oil as the main source of fat
- Small to modest amounts of dairy, eggs, fish, and poultry
- Fish and chicken are eaten more often than red meat
- Plant-based foods with little processing are the main focus
- Small to moderate amounts of wine can be drunk with meals.
- Fruit is often served for dinner instead of sweets

Every year, U.S. News and World Report ranks the best meals and the Mediterranean diet comes out on **top**. A group of experts rates different eating plans and famous diets based on things like how healthy they are, how well they work, and how simple they are to follow. A lot of health groups and doctors also say that the Mediterranean diet is one of the healthiest. So, does it live up to the good name it has?[180]
A large study from Spain in 2013 found that eating in a Mediterranean way cut the chance of heart disease by 28% to 30%. It's good for you even if you don't live near the Mediterranean. A study from 2013 followed 6,229 American women and men between the ages of 44 and 84 for 8 years, and the researchers from Johns Hopkins and others found that a Mediterranean-style diet, regular exercise, a healthy weight, and not smoking could protect against early heart disease, slow the buildup of plaque in artery walls, and lower the risk of dying young by 80%.[181]

Super foods[182]

There is no one food, not even a "superfood," that can give us all the nutrients, health benefits, and energy we need. That being said, there are some things that deserve extra attention. The nutrients in these

---

[180] American Heart Association - https://www.heart.org/en/healthy-living/healthy-eating/eat-smart/nutrition-basics/mediterranean-diet (Reviewed in January 2020)
[181] John Hopkins Medicine - https://www.hopkinsmedicine.org/health/wellness-and-prevention/take-your-diet-to-the-mediterranean (Accessed in May 2024)
[182] Harvard Health Publishing - https://www.health.harvard.edu/blog/10-superfoods-to-boost-a-healthy-diet-2018082914463 (Published in October 2022)

"superfoods" are very important and can give your meals and snacks extra energy and they can also help you eat healthier overall.

- **Berries**. Berries are naturally sweet and high in fiber. Their bright colors show that they are also high in vitamins and nutrients that fight disease. It is just as healthy to buy frozen berries when they are not in season.
- **Fish**. Protein and omega-3 fatty acids, which help keep your heart healthy, can be found in fish. You can buy fish that is fresh, frozen, or canned. Salmon, tuna cuts, mackerel, herring, trout, anchovies, and sardines are the fish that have the most omega-3s.
- **Leafy greens**. You can get a lot of vitamin A, vitamin C, and iron from dark leafy greens. They also have a lot of phytochemicals, which are chemicals made by plants that are good for your health. They also make you eat more fiber.
- **Nuts**. Peanuts, almonds, pecans, hazelnuts, and other nuts are good sources of plant protein. Also, they have polyunsaturated fats, which may help lower the risk of heart disease. But remember that they are high in calories, so don't eat more than a handful.
- **Olive oil**. A lot of vitamin E, polyphenols, and monounsaturated fatty acids can be found in olive oil. All of these help lower the chance of heart disease. Use instead of margarine or butter.
- **Whole grains**. Whole grains are a good source of both soluble and insoluble fiber. They also have a lot of minerals, phytonutrients, and B vitamins. It has been shown that they lower cholesterol and keep you from getting diabetes and heart disease. If you're at the store buying bread, make sure the first thing on the list is "100% whole wheat flour".
- **Yogurt**. Yogurt has probiotics, which are live bacteria. These "good bacteria" can keep the body safe from bacteria that are worse for it. It is a good source of calcium and protein. Eat more yogurt but be careful with fruit-flavored or flavored yogurts because they have a lot of extra sugar added to them. You can

add your own fruit to plain yogurt. In soups and dips, you can use yogurt instead of mayonnaise or sour cream.

- **Cruciferous vegetables**. Broccoli, cauliflower, cabbage, kohlrabi, radishes, turnips, collard greens, and mustard greens are some of these. These foods are full of fiber, vitamins, and phytochemicals like indoles, thiocyanates, and nitriles that may help fight some types of cancer.
- **Legumes**. Soybeans, peas, kidney beans, black beans, red beans, and garbanzo beans are all in this large group. You can get a lot of fiber, calcium, and plant-based protein from legumes. It has been shown that they can help lower the chance of getting heart disease.
- **Tomatoes**. These have a lot of lycopene and vitamin C, which lowers the risk of getting prostate cancer.

Becoming a vegetarian and vegan[183]

There are many **reasons** why people choose to be vegetarian, such as their health, their religious beliefs, their worry for animal welfare or the use of antibiotics and hormones in livestock, or their desire to eat in a way that doesn't harm the environment. It's possible for some people to not eat meat because they can't afford it. It's easier and more appealing to become a vegetarian now that fresh produce is available all year, there are more vegetarian restaurants, and food from countries that eat mostly plants is becoming more popular.

Traditionally, most research into vegetarianism was concerned with possible nutritional deficits, but recently the focus has shifted to the health benefits of a meat-free diet, and more and more studies are backing this up. These days, eating only plants is seen as not only **healthy**, but also a way to lower your risk of getting many long-term diseases. As per the US Dietetic Association, "appropriately planned vegetarian diets, including total vegetarian or vegan diets, are healthful,

---

[183] Harvard Health Publishing - https://www.health.harvard.edu/staying-healthy/becoming-a-vegetarian (Published in April 2020)

nutritionally adequate, and may provide health benefits in the prevention and treatment of certain diseases".

"**Appropriately planned**" is the key phrase. Becoming a vegetarian might not be good for you if you don't follow the rules for nutrition, fat intake, and weight control. After all, a diet of drinks, pizza with cheese, and candy is still "vegetarian". In order to stay healthy, you should eat a lot of different fruits, veggies, and whole grains. Good fats, like those in nuts, olive oil, and canola oil, should be used instead of heavy and trans fats. Always remember that you'll gain weight if you eat too many calories, even if they come from healthy, low-fat plant-based foods. For this reason, it's also important to watch your portions, read food labels, and stay active.

When compared to meat eaters, vegans tend to eat more fiber, folic acid, potassium, magnesium, and phytochemicals (plant chemicals) like carotenoids and flavonoids and less saturated fat and cholesterol. So, their total and LDL (bad) cholesterol, blood pressure, and body mass index (BMI) are likely to be lower. All of these things are linked to living longer and a lower chance of many chronic diseases. But we still don't have enough information to say for sure how a vegetarian diet affects health in the long run. It's hard to tell the difference between the effect of vegetarianism and other habits that vegetarians are more likely to have, like not smoking, not drinking too much, and exercising adequately.

You can change your diet to **be more vegetarian** even if you don't want to become a vegetarian. For example, you could eat more plant-based energy sources like tofu or beans or fish instead of meat a few times a week.

Vegetarians are people who don't eat any kind of meat or seafood, but there are a lot of different **types** of people who call themselves vegetarians, such as:

- If you are a **vegan** (a total vegetarian), you should not eat any animal products, like eggs, dairy, fish, meat, or poultry.
- **Lacto-ovo** vegetarians don't eat meat and fish, but they do eat eggs and things made from milk.

- **Lacto** vegetarians don't eat meat, fish, or eggs, but they do eat dairy products.
- People who are **ovo** vegetarians don't eat meat, fish, or dairy, but they do eat eggs.
- **Partially** vegetarians: they don't eat meat but can eat fish (pesco-vegetarian) or chicken (pollo-vegetarian).

Dietary supplements[184, 185]

At the grocery store near you, there are shelves full of bottles of vitamins. Minerals and vitamins from A to zinc are among these.
There are a lot of over-the-counter dietary supplements on the **market**. In the US alone, more than 90,000 items bring in about $30 billion a year.
A broad term for all kinds of supplements, from vitamins and minerals to herbs and biosimilars, is "dietary supplement". Most of the time, though, "supplement" refers to either a vitamin or mineral supplement or a multivitamin, which is a product that has 10 or more vitamins, minerals, or both.

Every day, we **need many nutrients** to stay healthy. For example, calcium and vitamin D protect our bones, folic acid helps our bodies make and keep new cells, and vitamin A keeps our immune systems and eyes healthy.
Supplements are popular, but there isn't much proof that they are actually good for your health. A study from the Journal of the American College of Cardiology in 2018, showed that multivitamins, vitamin D, calcium, and vitamin C—the four supplements that people most often take—did not protect against heart disease.
When people do things they think are good for them, they feel better.

---

[184] Harvard Health Publishing - https://www.health.harvard.edu/staying-healthy/do-you-need-a-daily-supplement (Published in February 2021)
[185] Harvard Health Publishing - https://www.health.harvard.edu/staying-healthy/dietary-supplements-do-they-help-or-hurt (Published in January 2013)

Supplements should never be used instead of a healthy, well-balanced diet, and they can even get in the way of healthy habits that are much more beneficial.

There are **no rules** about dietary supplements because they are not regulated by FDA as drugs, but foods. But a lot of dietary pills have ingredients that have strong biological effects that might not work well with a medicine you are on or a health problem you may have. Products that contain hidden drugs are sometimes sold as dietary supplements when they are not, which puts customers at even greater risk. Because of these things, you should talk to a doctor or nurse before taking any dietary product.
Supplements don't have to show that they're useful before they can be sold. Because there aren't many rules and regulations, it's also hard to be sure that the supplement has all the chemicals listed on the label and is free of any other substances that could be harmful.

In more thorough **research**, some products that were thought to be good for your health in observational studies were found to not only not work, but also be dangerous. At first, vitamin E was thought to be good for the heart, but later, it was found to raise the risk of bleeding strokes. Folic acid and other B vitamins used to be thought to help prevent heart disease and strokes, however, later studies not only didn't confirm that benefit, but they also raised concerns that high doses of these nutrients might raise the chance of cancer.
Many nutrients are bad for you when you eat too much of them, and they have something called an "upper intake level". Calcium, iron, zinc, vitamins A, B6, C, and D, as well as some minerals, have these limits. Getting more than that amount on a regular basis can be very bad for your health, and companies that make these supplements don't have to keep their goods below these upper limits.
A study from 2012 by Harvard called Physicians' Health Study II found that men who took a multivitamin every day for 11 years had an 8% lower risk of cancer and a 9% lower risk of cataracts than men who took a placebo (a pill that doesn't do anything). But, and this is a big but,

many of those interesting supplement studies were just that—observational. They didn't test one supplement against placebo in a controlled setting. Observational studies can't show that the treatment is what's good for your health because they can't fully control things like diet, exercise, and other factors.

Vitamin D should be brought up in particular. Direct sunlight on the skin outside makes vitamin D in the body, and most people should be able to get all the vitamin D they need from sunlight from late March or early April to the end of September.
But from October to early March, the sun doesn't give us enough vitamin D, while some foods also have vitamin D, it's hard to get enough vitamin D from food alone. Everyone, including women who are pregnant or breastfeeding, should think about taking a daily supplement with 10 micrograms of vitamin D in the fall and winter. The UK government advices so.[186]

For some high-risk **groups**, supplements can also be very helpful. For example, people who have been diagnosed with osteoporosis may need more calcium and vitamin D than they normally get from their food. Supplements can also help people who have Crohn's disease or celiac disease, which make it hard for their bodies to receive certain nutrients. People who don't eat certain things might also need more nutrients. Vitamin B12, for example, can only be found in animal goods, so if you are a vegan, you might not get enough B12 from the food you eat.
A mix of vitamin C, vitamin E, carotenoids, zinc, and copper has also been shown to slow down the progression of age-related macular degeneration, which is a major cause of vision loss in older people.
This is meant to show that taking vitamins as directed by a doctor can help people who have certain health problems. If not, it's better to get minerals and vitamins from food instead of pills.

---

[186] National Health Service - https://www.nhs.uk/conditions/vitamins-and-minerals/vitamin-d (Reviewed in August 2020)

Nutritional labeling

The **Nutri-Score** was created by French scientists and includes suggested parts like fiber and some proteins, along with the amount of sugar, fat, and salt. It only gives the food one value on a 5-point scale that goes from "A" on a dark green field for the best balance to a yellow "C" and a red "E" for the worst. A lot of research has shown that the Nutri-Score is the easiest way to understand nutrition labels and helps people pick goods that are better for them.

The International Agency for Research on Cancer (IARC), which is part of the World Health Organization (WHO), has asked the European Union commission to make the Nutri-Score a law in Europe. It would help people choose better foods, which is very important for stopping cancer and other long-term diseases that cause death.

At the moment, countries in the **European Union** like France, Belgium, Spain, Switzerland, Germany, Luxembourg, and the Netherlands use the Nutri-Score method on a voluntary basis.

Some people say that the system may favor highly processed foods that aren't very good for you while lowering the value of natural, organic, and regional goods because of its methodological flaws. The method is not meant to be used to compare the nutritional value of different types of food, therefore people may not understand the information on product packages if they don't know this.[187]

The **traffic light** method on food labels in the **UK** tells you whether a food has a lot or a little of fat, saturated fat, sugar, and salt. In addition, it will tell you how many calories and kilojoules are in that item. As you can see from the color-coded sticker, green means the food is low in a certain nutrient, amber means it is medium, and red means it is high in that nutrient.[188]

---

[187] Foodwatch - https://www.foodwatch.org/en/who-eu-wide-introduction-of-nutri-score-necessary (Published in September 2021)

[188] Food Standard Agency - https://www.food.gov.uk/safety-hygiene/check-the-label (Accessed in May 2024)

Labels in the **US** might not be as eye-catching as the ones presented before, but they are still as informative. It uses an easy table to show how much of the "Big Three" (sodium, sugar, and saturated fat) these foods contain. These can affect our weight and blood pressure, which can raise the risk of heart disease and stroke.

Genetically Modified Organisms (GMOs)[189]

Genetically Modified Organisms, or GMOs, are living things (like plants, animals, or microorganisms) whose DNA has been changed in a way that doesn't happen normally when species mate and their DNA combines with each other. "**Gene technology**" or "modern biotechnology" are other names for this technique, and it lets certain genes move from one living thing to another, even if the two species are not connected.
GM foods are made and sold because they are thought to be good for either the people who make them or the people who eat them. This should lead to a product that is either cheaper or better in some way, like lasting longer or having more nutrients.

The main goal of the GM crops that are currently on the market is to **protect crops** better by making them resistant to plant diseases caused by insects or viruses or by making them more tolerant of pesticides. As a consequence, the amount of pesticides used has gone down in places where there are a lot of weeds because of these crops.

To make sure that GM organisms and foods are **safe** for people and the environment, certain processes have been set up just for that purpose, while most of the time, similar tests are not done on regular foods. The safety tests for the GM foods that are currently on the foreign market have been passed, and they are not likely to be harmful to people's health. These foods have also been shown to have no negative effects on human health when eaten by the general public in the countries where they are legal. Making sure GM foods are safe should start with

---

[189] Food and Drugs Administration - https://www.fda.gov/food/food-new-plant-varieties/understanding-new-plant-varieties (Accessed in May 2024)

regular safety checks based on the Codex Alimentarius guidelines and, if needed, proper tracking after the food has been sold.

Water, essence of life[190]

Water is an essential part of the human body, forming more than half of it.

Water makes up different **amounts of body mass** in different people. Babies have the most, with about 78% when they are born, and that number drops to about 65% by the time the child is 1 year old. About 60% of a grown man's body is water. Lean tissue, on the other hand, has more water than fat tissue, so this means that people with more fat tissue have less water than people with less fat tissue. For this reason, about 55% of an adult woman's body is water because she generally has more fat than a man.

One of the most important parts of the diet is **staying hydrated**. Making sure you drink enough liquids to keep your body's fluid levels up helps make sure that all of its processes can happen normally. Fluids in the body are necessary for many things to happen, like the blood bringing glucose, oxygen, and nutrients to cells and the kidneys getting rid of waste. It also keeps our skin healthy, helps our digestive system work, and keeps our eyes and joints smooth.

Our bodies are specially made to keep their temperature stable. When it's hot, for example, we lose more water through our skin (perspiration), which cools the body and helps keep the temperature stable.

Drinking water is important for people of all ages, but it's especially important for older people.

Headaches, dizziness, tiredness, trouble focusing, and a dry mouth can all be caused by not drinking enough water. Long-term, not drinking enough water can make you constipated and add to your risk of getting urinary tract infections and kidney stones.

---

[190] British Dietetic Association - https://www.bda.uk.com/resource/the-importance-of-hydration.html (Published in August 2019)

Adults should drink between **1.5 and 2 liters of water every day**. Most mugs and glasses hold 200 milliliters, which is 8 to 10 drinks a day. Kids don't need as many drinks as adults do, and they should aim for about 6 to 8 drinks a day. But by the time they are teens, their needs are the same as adults'.
More water needs to be replaced when we sweat, so people who live in hot places or who sweat more while playing sports will need to drink more water more often to make up for what they lose through sweating. Waiting until you feel thirsty is not a good enough sign that you need to drink, because by the time we feel thirsty, our bodies are already dehydrated and may be feeling some of the effects. In the same way, drinking just to quench your thirst does not fully refresh the body. The color of your pee is the best way to tell if you're properly hydrated. A pale straw-colored urine is a good sign, but if your pee is darker, it means your body needs more water.
To put it simply, any drink will help you stay hydrated, so we can also count other drinks as part of our overall fluid intake. Since milk, fruit juice, tea, coffee, and soft drinks are all mostly water, they can be counted.
A little over 20% to 30% of the fluids we eat and drink come from food. The water content of many fruits and veggies, like cucumbers, tomatoes, melons, and courgettes, is over 90%, so these foods help us stay hydrated.

It is very important for **athletes** to drink enough water because they lose more water through sweating when they work out. It is well known that athletes can lose efficiency if they don't drink enough water. Isotonic sports drinks are often used by athletes to recover the salts and water they lose when they sweat. In fact, drinking every day is just as much a part of their training as what they eat and how strong they are. On the other side, most of us who only play sports occasionally, go to the gym, or run for fun don't need the more expensive sports drinks. Instead, we should only drink water to stay hydrated.

Tap or bottled water?[191]

The water in your **tap** comes from big lakes, rivers, wells, or storage tanks, and before this water is pumped into homes and businesses, it usually goes through a water treatment plant.

In some places, dirty drinking water is a problem, but tap water is usually safe, easy to get, and good for the earth.

The Centers for Disease Control and Prevention (CDC) say that the water in the United States is one of the best in the world. Environmental Protection Agency (EPA) rules govern public tap water in the United States, and it has set legal limits on more than 90 contaminants right now, including heavy metals like lead and bacteria like Escherichia coli (E. coli). Even so, pollution of drinking water can still happen, and old plumbing can introduce contaminants like lead, and natural disasters like floods can briefly make public water systems dirty. A lot of groups that work to protect public health also say that the EPA's rules aren't strict enough on some toxins.

The Environmental Working Group (EWG) says that the rules about water in the United States haven't been changed in almost 20 years, so, some chemicals may be hurting people who are already weak, like children and women who are pregnant.

On top of that, house water filters might make your tap water safer.

The best things about tap water might be how cheap and easy it is to get.

Some people think that **bottled** water is safer, tastes better, and is easier to get than tap water, but there are some worries about its safety and effect on the environment.

A lot of people say that bottled water tastes better than tap water, but most people can't tell the difference between the two in random taste tests.

---

[191] HealthLine - https://www.healthline.com/nutrition/tap-water-vs-bottled-water (Published in June 2020)

Even though bottled water is sometimes recalled because it has contaminants, it is usually thought to be safe, but some items may have microplastics, which are very small pieces of plastic.
Animal studies and other research show that microplastics are chemicals that mess with hormones, cause inflammation, hurt health, and build up over time in organs like the liver, kidneys, and bowels.
In 2018, 11 popular bottled water brands from 9 countries were tested, and 93% of the 259 bottles that were looked at found microplastics. Part of this pollution came from the way the bottles were packed and the bottling process itself.

Eating disorders[192]

A common misunderstanding is that people with eating problems choose to live this way, however eating disorders are serious illnesses that can be **fatal**. They cause people to have major problems with their eating habits, as well as their thoughts and feelings about food. An eating problem may also be shown by being obsessed with food, weight, or shape.
Some common eating disorders are:

- **Anorexia nervosa**: This is a situation in which a person either doesn't eat at all or eats very little of only certain foods. They may also weigh themselves repeatedly because they might think they are overweight even if they are dangerously underweight. Anorexia nervosa can end in death, and if you compare its death rate to that of other mental illnesses, it is very high. People who have anorexia are more likely to die from health problems that come with being hungry and by suicide.
- **Bulimia nervosa** is a disorder in which people eat abnormally large amounts of food over and over again and feel powerless to stop these episodes. After binge-eating, the person does something to make up for it, like forcing themselves to vomit,

[192] National Institute of Mental Health - https://www.nimh.nih.gov/health/topics/eating-disorders (Reviewed in January 2023)

using too much laxatives or diuretics, fasting, working out too much, or a mix of these things.

- **Binge-eating disorder**: Binge-eating disorder is a mental illness in which people lose control of their eating and eat a lot of food at once. People who binge-eat don't purge, work out too much, or go without food afterward like people with bulimia nervosa do. People who have binge-eating problems are often overweight or obese because of this. In the U.S., binge-eating disorder is the most common type of eating disorder.

People of all ages, races or ethnicities, weights, and genders can have eating disorders. People with eating disorders often start showing symptoms in their teens or early 20s, but they can also start showing symptoms in childhood or later in life.

Scientists have found that genetic, biological, behavioral, psychological, and social **factors** all work together to cause eating problems, and new science and technology are being used by researchers to learn more about eating problems.

People with eating problems should get help as soon as possible, since people who have eating issues are more likely to commit suicide and have health problems. A lot of the time, people who have eating disorders also have other mental illnesses, like anxiety or sadness, or do drugs. It is possible to fully heal from these disorders.

Physical activity

All kinds of movement are considered physical exercise, such as sports, cycling, wheeling, walking, active recreation, and play. No matter how good you are at it, anyone can do it for fun.
The Latin **word** for "muscle" means "little mouse," which is what the Romans thought stretched bicep muscles looked like.[193]

Much of the world is becoming **less active**. The amount of inaction rises as a country's economy grows, and these numbers can be as high as 70% in some countries because of changes in transportation, more people using technology, cultural values, and more people living in cities.[194]
About 110,000 deaths a year could be avoided if people in the US aged 40 and up did a little more moderate to vigorous physical exercise. It would help to work out for even 10 minutes longer every day.
Taking more steps every day can also help lower the risk of dying too soon from any cause. For adults younger than 60, the chance of dying too soon stopped rising after about 8,000 to 10,000 steps per day, and for people 60 and older after about 6,000 to 8,000 steps per day.[195]

Regular physical activity **helps** in many ways:

- Managing your **weight**: what you eat and how much you exercise are both very important.
- **Cardiovascular disease**: If you do at least 150 minutes of mild exercise a week, you may be less likely to get these diseases, since being active on a regular basis can also drop your blood

---

[193] Oxford English Dictionary - https://www.oed.com/dictionary/muscle_n?tl=true&tab=etymology (Accessed in May 2024)
[194] World Health Organization - https://www.who.int/initiatives/sports-and-health (Accessed in May 2024)
[195] Centers for Disease Control and Prevention - https://www.cdc.gov/physicalactivity/basics/pa-health/index.htm (Reviewed in August 2023)

pressure and raise your HDL. You can lower your risk even more by being active more often.

- **Type 2 Diabetes and Metabolic Syndrome**: If you work out regularly, you may be less likely to get type 2 diabetes and metabolic syndrome. When you have metabolic syndrome, you have high blood sugar, too much fat around your waist, low HDL cholesterol, high lipids, or high blood pressure. Amounts of physical activity tend to help people even if they don't meet the guidelines of 150 minutes of moderate physical activity a week.
- **Infectious diseases**: Being active may lower the chance of getting complications from infectious illnesses like COVID-19, the flu, and pneumonia.
- **Cancers**: Being active lowers your chance of getting a number of common cancers. Being physically active lowers an adult's risk of getting cancer in the bladder, breast, colon, endometrial, esophagus, kidney, lung, or stomach.

  Getting regular exercise is also good for people who have survived cancer because it makes them healthier and lowers their risk of getting another cancer.
- **Muscles and bones**: As you get older, it's important to take care of your muscles, joints, and bones because they support your body and help you move. Lifting weights and other muscle-strengthening exercises can help you gain or keep muscle mass and strength, and this is important for older people whose muscle mass and power decrease as they age. No matter what age you are, slowly raising the weight and number of reps you do to strengthen your muscles will give you even more benefits.
- **Daily Activities**: Some everyday activities are going up and down stairs, doing grocery shopping, or playing with your grandkids. A functional restriction means not being able to do normal things. People in their middle or older years who are physically active are less likely to have problems with their daily lives than people who are not active. Different kinds of physical exercise help older people's bodies work better and lower their risk of falling and getting hurt. A hip fracture is a very bad injury that can

happen after falling, and if you're an older adult, breaking your hip can change your whole life for the worse.

- **Mental health**: Being active on a regular basis can help you think, learn, and make decisions as you get older. You may also feel less depressed and anxious, and it may help you sleep better.
- **Chronic illnesses and disabilities**: daily exercise can help people with long-term illnesses and disabilities deal with them. Regular exercise can help adults with arthritis feel less pain and improve their function, mood, and quality of life. It can also help people with type 2 diabetes control their blood sugar levels and lower their risk of heart disease and nerve damage. Finally, it can help people with disabilities do daily tasks and stay independent.

Sports injuries[196]

"Sports injury" refers to the types of injuries that most often happen during exercise or sports, but they **don't just happen to athletes**. People who work in factories get tennis elbows, artists get shoulder injuries, and gardeners get tendinitis, even if they don't play sports.

There are two main types of sports injuries: **acute** and **chronic** injuries. Acute injuries happen quickly, like when someone falls, gets hit, or twists a joint. Chronic injuries, on the other hand, are usually caused by overusing one part of the body and get worse over time. Ankle sprains and dislocations are examples of short-term injuries, while shin splints and stress fractures are examples of long-term injuries.

Sports injuries are **handled** in different ways, but most minor ones can be taken care of at home by Resting, Icing, Compressing, and Elevating (**R-I-C-E**) the hurt area. People with more serious injuries need to see a doctor. They may set you up with physical therapy to help you heal

---

[196] National Institute of Arthritis and Musculoskeletal and Skin Diseases - https://www.niams.nih.gov/health-topics/sports-injuries (Accessed in May 2024)

and/or fit you for a cast, splint, or brace, and there are times when you might need surgery. Before going back to the sport or activity that hurt you, you should generally go through a rehabilitation program that includes exercise and other types of therapy.

Bad things can happen when you work out or play sports, but most physical exercise is safe for most people, and the health benefits are much greater than the risks.

The **risk factors** for sports injuries include:

- Not doing **correctly** the exercises
- **Overtraining**, which means working out too much, too often, or for too long.
  When you don't give your muscles enough time to heal between workouts, you overdo it and end up with sore muscles that are worse than usual. Overtraining usually happens after a few days of hard training in a row, which makes you feel tired. Luckily, resting is an easy way to undo the effects of overextending yourself.
  Many players think that when they are weak or don't do well, it means they need to work out even harder, so they keep pushing themselves, and this makes the body even worse. Overtraining can make it hard to fully heal, and you may need to stop working out for weeks or months. This can be especially hard for someone whose life revolves around their sport. Sleep, diet, and mental health are all very important for keeping you from overtraining.
- Increasing or decreasing the level of physical action **too quickly**
- When you play the **same sport** all year
- When you run or jump on **hard surfaces**: when you hit something hard, like asphalt, you could get hurt. For example, you could get shin pain or a stress fracture. It should be clear, flat, even, and pretty soft to run or jump on. Stay away from rough areas, sand, and concrete. Slowly introduce changes to the surface.

- Not putting on the **right gear**: a lot of games and exercises need some kind of gear, like shoes, bikes, or racquets. Wearing protective gear like mouthguards, shin pads, and helmets can greatly lower the chance of getting hurt by absorbing the force of falls or crashes. If you're using hand-held sports gear, make sure you have the right grip. For example, holding a tennis stick the wrong way can make you more likely to get tennis elbow (tendonitis). Make sure your gear fits your sport or activity, as well as your height, weight, and age. Protective gear should be worn during training as well as games and competitions. Lastly, keep an eye on your gear and change it when it gets worn out. Talk to your coach or the sports organization if you don't know how to check or keep your gear.
- Having been **hurt before**
- Having certain **anatomical features** that are unique to each joint or not being able to bend or stretch properly
- Taking certain **drugs**, like fluoroquinolones, a type of antibiotic that has been linked to tendinitis and tendon tears

Majority of injuries are caused by minor **trauma** involving muscles, ligaments, tendons, or bones, including:[197]

- **Contusions**, or bruises, are damages to soft tissue.
- **Sprains**: A sprain is when a ligament gets stretched or torn. Ligaments are fiber-filled bands that can bend and link bones to each other and to cartilage. They also keep your joints' bones together. Sprains most often happen in the wrists, ankles, or knees.
- **Strains**: A strain is when a muscle or tendon twists, pulls, or tears. This can happen because of too much use, force, or pulling. A tendon is a tough string of tissue that joins bones to muscles.

---

[197] Johns Hopkins Medicine - https://www.hopkinsmedicine.org/health/conditions-and-diseases/sports-injuries (Accessed in May 2024)

- **Fractures**: These are breaks in the bone that are usually caused by a fall or blow. A simple hairline fracture is a thin break that may not go all the way through the bone. A complex fracture is when the broken bone sticks out through the skin. Broken bones most often happen in the arms and legs.
- **Stress fractures** are weak spots or small cracks in the bone that happen because of overuse over time. People who train for dancing, running, and other sports often get stress fractures in their feet or legs. Runners are more likely to get stress fractures in the bones in the middle of their foot called metatarsals.
- **Dislocations**: A dislocation happens when a ligament is put under a lot of stress, letting the ends of two bones that are joined move apart. When joint muscles are under a lot of stress, the joint can move out of place.

How can I prevent a sports injury?[198]

The following are some basic steps to prevent a sports injury:

- Make **goals** that are realistic. Whether you want to swim more laps, lift more weight, or run a certain distance, make a goal that you can reach and then work to get better over time.
- Make **plans** and get ready: Come up with a workout plan that includes flexibility, strength training, and cardio. This will make it less likely that you will get hurt. Also, work out different muscle groups every other day and every other week, and spend some time learning the right way to do things for your sport or program. Getting a personal trainer or signing up for a class are often fun and safe ways to start something new. Wear shoes that support your feet and may fix some problems with your feet that can cause injuries, and make sure you have the right gear.

---

[198] Johns Hopkins Medicine - https://www.hopkinsmedicine.org/health/conditions-and-diseases/sports-injuries/preventing-sports-injuries (Accessed in May 2024)

- **Don't rush**; take your time. It takes time to get in shape or learn a new sport. It's important to give our bodies enough time to get used to the stresses that higher levels of training put on their bones, joints, and muscles. For example, if you want to run, slowly add more miles, and make sure you have plenty of time to rest between workouts. If you do get hurt while playing sports, make sure you get enough rest before doing any hard activities again.
- **Pay attention** to your body. If your body tells you it's under too much stress, change what you're doing. A mild muscle pain that doesn't last long is usually thought of as "good pain", but joint pain is not normal and means you should slow down.
- Drink plenty of **water**. To avoid dehydration, heat fatigue, and heatstroke, drink water.
- **Warm up and cool down**: Research has shown that muscles are less likely to get stressed when they are warm. This is why it is important to warm up before you work out. That's why you should do some light running or walking before you work out and again afterward to help your muscles cool down slowly. Getting more flexible is another important way to keep from getting hurt. To do this, stretch before and after a workout, but it's best to do it when the body is already warm.

The importance of stretching[199]

You might think that runners and dancers are the only ones who stretch. That being said, we all need to stretch to keep our freedom and movement.

A great many people don't know how **important** it is to stretch regularly, and you should do it **every day**.

Muscles need to be flexible, strong, and healthy to keep the joints moving freely. Stretching helps keep muscles flexible, strong, and healthy, otherwise they get short and tight. When you then ask the

[199] Harvard Health Publishing - https://www.health.harvard.edu/staying-healthy/the-importance-of-stretching (Published in March 2022)

muscles to do something, they are weak and can't reach their full length, and that makes you more likely to hurt your muscles, joints, or strains.

Since your body is full of muscles, the thought of stretching every day might be too much for you, but you don't have to stretch every muscle. Your calves, hamstrings, hip flexors in the pelvis, and quadriceps in the front of the thigh are the most important parts of your lower body for movement. It's also good for you to stretch your shoulders, neck, and lower back. You should try to stretch every day or at least 3 times a week.

You won't be completely flexible just because you stretched once today, because this is something you'll have to do **over time** and keep at it. Your muscles may not be completely flexible after just 1 or 2 lessons because it may take you months to get them that way.

In the past, we thought that stretching was important to get our muscles warmed up and ready for the activity. However, more and more studies have shown that stretching muscles before they're warm can hurt them. The fibers aren't ready when they are cold, and they could get damaged. To make the tissue more flexible and easier to change, **warm up first**, and this will bring blood to the area. 5 to 10 minutes of light movement, like a quick walk, is all it takes to get the muscles ready to stretch. Stretching can also be done after an aerobics or weights class.

Tend to stretch for one minute. Don't bounce because it can hurt you. While you stretch, you might feel tight, but it shouldn't hurt. If it does, don't stretch that muscle any further until you see a doctor.

The best sports and exercises[200]

In the United States, **running** is one of the most popular ways to stay fit. A 2010 study in Current Sports Medicine Reports, on the other hand, found that up to half of all runners get hurt every year.

---

[200] Time - https://time.com/5645509/healthiest-sports (Published in August 2019)

Also, a lot of runners do too much. Researchers have found that the best way to get the benefits of running for longer life is to do it 2 or 3 times a week at a slow to moderate pace.

If you are 40 or older, you are more likely to hurt your knees, shoulders, and other joints when you do **workouts that put a lot of stress** on them. Some examples are soccer, basketball, tennis, and other games where you have to jump, twist, or change directions quickly. That doesn't mean that these things are bad for you or that people who like them should stop doing them. A study published in 2018 in the journal Mayo Clinic Proceedings found that activities that involve spending time with other people are linked to longer life rates than activities that you do by yourself. Studies have separately linked both exercise and social interaction with living longer, so it makes sense that doing both together would be good. But even though many of these things are good for you, they also pose a high chance of injury.

Walking, swimming, and yoga are all low-risk, high-reward activities that people can do to lower their risks while still getting all the health and life benefits of exercise.
Swimming is a great way to get fit and stronger because it mixes aerobic exercise with resistance training.
A 2011 study in BMJ Open found that walking is linked to both a longer life and a lower chance of needing medical care. A 2019 study found that walking quickly is very good for you.
Yoga is a great way to get stronger and more flexible at the same time.

There are ways for exercise fans who don't want to live a life of long walks and yoga to lower their risk of getting hurt while still doing intense, high-impact sports.
Some people might yawn at the first tip. To avoid getting hurt, though, experts say to play sports or work out in a modest way. A lot of accidents happen when people train too much. Every day, you should not play the same sport or do the same kind of exercise, especially if you are pushing yourself very hard.

And finally, one more safety step is to start out slowly and work your way up to harder workouts. A lot of people begin with too much weight or volume. To build your strength and endurance, don't just sign up for this year's half-marathon but consider the one next year, and mix it with other types of exercise like swimming and yoga.
Finally, don't forget about your core. **Core strength** is important because if it's weak, you might use your arms or legs too much, making them hurt. You can get stronger in your core by taking **pilates** classes, and **machines** at the gym that work your upper and lower back, obliques, and abdominal muscles can do the same.

Boost your energy naturally[201]

You could feel tired **sometimes**, but it can be wrong if you always are.
If you've been tired for a few weeks and don't know why, if your tiredness gets in the way of your daily life, if you're lost weight or your mood changes, or if someone tells you that you make gasping, snorting, or choking sounds when you sleep, you should see a doctor.

Luckily, there are **things you can** do to make your own energy levels higher:

- Deal with your **stress**: Feelings that are caused by stress use up a lot of energy. Stress can be eased by talking to a friend or family member, joining a support group, or seeing a doctor. Meditation, self-hypnosis, yoga, and tai chi are all good examples of relaxation techniques that can help you feel less stressed.
- **Lighten up**: Being too tired is often caused by too much work. Professional, family, and social responsibilities can all add up to too much work. Your list of "must-do" things should be streamlined. Make a list of the most important things you need to do and cut down on the ones that aren't as important. If you need it, you might want to ask for more help at work.

---

[201] Harvard Health Publishing - https://www.health.harvard.edu/energy-and-fatigue/9-tips-to-boost-your-energy-naturally (Published in April 2024)

- **Work out**: Working out almost promises that you'll sleep better. It also moves air around your body and gives your cells more energy to burn. Also, working out can raise the amount of dopamine in your brain, which can help improve your happiness. If you want to get even more health benefits from walking, speed up every once in a while.
- **Do not smoke**. You already know that smoking is bad for your health. But you might not know that smoking drains your energy by making you sleepless. Nicotine in tobacco is a stimulant, which speeds up the heart rate, raises blood pressure, and makes it harder to fall asleep by activating brain waves that are linked to being awake. If you do fall asleep, the drug's ability to make you want it again once you wake up.
- Get **less sleep**: If you think you might not be getting enough sleep, try getting less sleep. It might sound strange, but figuring out how much sleep you really need can help you sleep better when you're in bed. In the long run, this process helps you sleep better and makes it easier to fall asleep. To do it do not take naps during the day and spend less time in bed the first night and only sleep for 4 hours. If you think you slept well during those 4 hours, sleep an extra 15 to 30 minutes the next night. You can slowly add more sleep each night as long as you're sleeping well the whole time you're in bed.
- Fuel up with **food**: mostly with food that has a low glycemic index, which means their sugars are absorbed slowly. This may help you escape the energy dip that usually happens after eating refined starches or sugars that are absorbed quickly. Whole grains, veggies high in fiber, nuts, and healthy oils like olive oil are all foods with a low glycemic index. In general, foods that are high in carbohydrates have the highest glycemic scores. There is almost no glucose index in proteins and fats.
- Make the most of **caffeine**. Coffee can help you focus because caffeine makes you more alert, but if you want coffee to wake you up, you have to use it wisely. It can keep you up at night, especially if you drink a lot of it or after 2 p.m. Most of the time,

tea gives less energy than coffee. The USDA's Food Data Central database says that an 8-ounce (230 milliliters) cup of home-brewed coffee has about 92 milligrams of caffeine, while a 12-ounce (350 milliliters) serving of coffee from a coffee shop has about 150 to 235 mg. On the other side, 8 ounces of black tea has about 47 milligrams of caffeine, and 8 ounces of green tea 29 milligrams of caffeine. Coffee may give you a quick boost of energy because it has a lot of caffeine, but tea has L-theanine, a chemical that, when mixed with caffeine, can help you stay mentally alert for longer. To put it another way, coffee gives you a quick and strong boost, but tea may give you a slower, steadier boost. The Food and Drug Administration says that most people can safely consume up to 400 milligrams of caffeine per day, and it may even be good for them, since caffeine can give you more energy and help you concentrate, and in small amounts, it may also lower your chance of depression, Parkinson's disease, liver fibrosis, heart disease, and some cancers. On the other hand, too much caffeine can make you antsy, nervous, or jittery. Using too much the stimulant can also be dangerous.[202]

- Drinking less **booze** is one of the best ways to avoid getting down in the middle of the afternoon, because at noon, alcohol is especially likely to make you sleepy. In the same way, if you want to be energetic in the evening, don't drink a cocktail at 5 o'clock. If you're going to drink, do it in balance and when you don't mind letting down your guard.
- Drink **water**. What is the only nutrient that has been shown to improve ability in most endurance sports? It's not a fancy sports drink, that's water. One of the first signs that your body needs more water is feeling tired.

There are a lot of vitamins, herbs, and other products in stores that claim to give you more energy. Some are put in soft drinks and other

[202] Forbes - https://www.forbes.com/health/nutrition/coffee-vs-tea (Updated in September 2023)

food as well. But there isn't much or any scientific proof that ginseng, guarana (which is another source of caffeine and is sometimes called Brazilian cocoa), and chromium picolinate really work.

Energy drinks are often advertised as goods that give you more energy, make you smarter, and improve your physical and mental performance. Energy drinks are the second most popular dietary supplement among teens and young people in the United States, after multivitamins. A big part of them is caffeine, and they might also have guarana, sugars, taurine, ginseng, and B vitamins in them.
There is more and more scientific proof that energy drinks are bad for your health, especially for kids, teens, and young adults. Several studies have shown that energy drinks make people stronger and more durable, but there is less proof that they have any effect on muscle strength or power. Energy drinks might make you more alert and help you react faster, but they might also make your hands less stable.
Energy drinks have a wide range of caffeine amounts, and it may not be easy to figure out how much caffeine is in a drink. A lot of caffeine can be bad for your heart and blood vessels, since it can mess up your heartbeat and make your heart rate and blood pressure go up. Caffeine may also be bad for kids whose heart and nervous systems are still growing. People who drink a lot of caffeine may also have problems with nervousness, sleep, digestion, and staying hydrated. Drinking too many energy drinks may make it harder for teens to sleep and may be linked to more risky behavior.[203]

---

[203] National Center For Complementary and Alternative Medicine - https://www.nccih.nih.gov/health/energy-drinks (Updated in July 2018)

Accidents and poisoning

"The ideal man bears the accidents of life with dignity and grace, making the best of the circumstances"
Aristotele (Greek philosopher and polymath, 350 BC)

More Americans die in the first half of their lives from injuries and violence than from any other cause, like cancer, HIV, or the flu. Examples include car accidents, suicides, and murders.

These are the **top 10 leading causes of death** in the U.S. for **ages 1-44** in 2020[204]:

- Unintentional injury 80.2k
- Suicide: 22.4k
- Homicide: 18.8k
- Heart disease: 17.3k
- Malignant cancer: 16.7k
- COVID-19: 8.9k
- Liver disease: 6.62k
- Diabetes: 4.45k
- Stroke: 2.93k
- Influenza and pneumonia: 2.1k

Also, in 2020, unintended injuries took away more **years of possible life** than any other cause of death.
If someone dies too soon (before age 65), the number of years of possible life lost is an estimate of how many more years they would have lived.
On these accidents, the split reason is shown below, along with the number of years of possible life lost for each[205]:

- Poisoning: 1.970k
- Motor Vehicle Traffic: 922k
- Drowning: 116k
- Suffocation: 107k
- Falls: 72k
- Other injuries: 216k

---

[204] Centers for Disease Control and Prevention - https://www.cdc.gov/injury/wisqars/animated-leading-causes.html (Reviewed in February 2022)
[205] Centers for Disease Control and Prevention - https://www.cdc.gov/injury/wisqars/fatal/index.html (Accessed in May 2024)

Poisoning[206]

Poisoning is a big problem in the US; it's the main reason people die from accidental injuries, even more than car accidents.
Exposures in childhood often happen because of kids' natural curiosity. In these situations, the amounts eaten are generally small, but even small amounts of some drugs and household chemicals can make kids very sick or even kill them.

Adult poisonings, on the other hand, are usually caused by **drugs**. They can be overdoses of illegal drugs or legal drugs taken for reasons other than medical ones, or in the wrong dose, or side effects from prescription drugs.
Within the past few years, more people have died from prescription painkillers like oxycodone, hydrocodone, and methadone than from heroin and coke put together. There will be a part in the end of this book just about drugs.

Pesticides, cleaning products, personal care and topical products, and other household items are some of the 10 most poisonous chemicals that people are exposed to every year. Poisons at work can happen from a number of different chemicals.

In the United States, **carbon monoxide (CO)** pollution kills more people than any other substance. CO is a poisonous gas that has no color or smell and is made when fuels burn incompletely. That's right—84% of the CO in the air comes from outside sources, with 59% coming from cars and trucks and 25% coming from lawnmowers, building equipment, airplanes, boats, and trains. CO poisonings, on the other hand, mostly happen in the home (73% of the time) from sources that aren't properly kept or vented inside or near the home.

---

[206] Centers for Disease Control and Prevention - https://www.cdc.gov/pictureofamerica/pdfs/picture_of_america_poisoning.pdf (Accessed in May 2024)

A lot of CO poisoning happens in the winter and during bad weather (like hurricanes, snowstorms, and blizzards) because people use their heaters and portable generators more. Low levels of CO exposure can make you tired and give you flu-like symptoms like headaches, nausea, and vomiting. High levels of CO exposure can make you lose your balance, fall, go into a coma, stop your heart and lungs from working, and even kill you. Up to 15% to 49% of people who survive a CO poisoning end up with long-term health problems, such as memory loss and problems with higher-order cognitive processing, which makes it harder to set goals, plan, organize, react appropriately, and keep an eye on oneself.

To avoid getting carbon monoxide poisoning, you can do certain things.

- Professionally **repair** your heating systems, water heaters, and any other gas, oil, or coal-burning appliances in the late summer or early fall.
- Put in CO **detectors** that run on batteries in your houses. Every spring and fall, when you change the clocks, check, or replace the batteries. If a device sounds, you should leave the house right away and call the emergency number.
- Get **medical help** right away if you think you might have CO poisoning and feel sick, dizzy, or lightheaded.
- **Never use** a generator, charcoal grill, camp stove, or any other engine that burns gasoline or charcoal inside the house, in the basement, in the garage, or outside the house near a window.
- Even if the **garage door** is open, you should never leave a car or truck running in a garage that is connected to a house.
- If your **stove or furnace** doesn't have a way for air to get out, don't use it. Also, don't use a gas oven for heat.

Car accidents[207]

Worldwide, about 1.3 million people lose their lives every year in car accidents, plus 20 to 50 million more people are hurt but don't die, and many of them become disabled because of their injury.
Road traffic injuries are the **8th leading cause of death** for all age groups and the leading cause of death for children and young adults aged 5-29 years.
More than half of all traffic deaths happen to people who are weak on the road, like walkers, cyclists, and motorcyclists.
It is interesting that 93% of road deaths happen in low- and middle-income countries, even though these countries have about 60% of the world's cars.
As early as elementary school, boys are more likely than girls to be in car accidents, and 73% of all traffic deaths are men younger than 25. Young males are almost 3 times more likely to die in a traffic accident than young females.

Typical **risk factors** are:

- **Speeding**: The chances of a crash happening and how bad the damage from the crash is both directly linked to the average speed. In this case, the risk of a fatal crash goes up by 4% for every 1% increase in mean speed and the risk of a major crash goes up by 3% for every 1% increase in mean speed.
- **Drinking** and other **drugs** that make you feel high: Between 5% and 35% of all traffic deaths are thought to be caused by drinking. For drunk driving, the chance of an accident starts to rise at low Blood Alcohol Concentrations (BAC) and gets much higher when the driver's BAC is ≥ 0.04 g/dl.
- Not using **safety equipment**: wearing a helmet correctly can cut the risk of fatal injuries by 42%. Also, wearing a seat belt lowers the risk of death by 45 to 50% for people in the front seats, and

[207] World Health Organization - https://www.who.int/news-room/fact-sheets/detail/road-traffic-injuries (Published in June 2022)

by 25% for people in the back seats. People who use child restraints are 60% less likely to die.

Nils Bohlin, an engineer at Volvo, came up with the current three-point seat belt in 1959. The company chose to leave the patent open, so all car companies could use the design for free, even though it was protected by a patent. The choice to make this rather unusual move was made to improve public safety so that everyone, whether they drove a Volvo or not, could be safer in traffic. A new idea that helped save more than a million lives.

- **Distracted driving**: There are many types of distractions that can make it hard to drive, but cell phones are becoming a bigger problem for road safety. About 4 times as many accidents happen to drivers who are on their phones as to drivers who are not on their phones. Hands-free phones are not much safer than hand-held phone sets, and texting makes the chance of an accident much higher.

First aid

Several thousand people die or are badly hurt in accidents every year, and many of these **deaths could be avoided** if first aid was given before the emergency arrived.

If we see someone hurt and in need of medical help right away, our first instinct is to give them what they need.

First aid is the immediate medical care that is given to anyone who is sick or hurt, no matter how bad their illness is, to save their life until help or an ambulance comes. This is very important to keep things from getting worse and to help the person who was hurt get better quickly.

For first aid, you don't always need a professional, trained person, or certain tools and supplies, since it can even be done by someone who is aware of their surroundings and doesn't have any special tools.

In some circumstances, first aid is the only care an injured person might need, while in other cases, it may be required to keep the patient alive till paramedics or an ambulance arrive to transfer him to a competent facility for further treatment. Official first aid training is the best way to

handle these situations, but until then, it's helpful to know some basic skills and techniques that can save lives.
Remember to stay calm, watch out for danger, and never put your own safety at risk.

Check, Call, Care[208]

Check: first, check if the person is responsive. Would they like your help? If the person can't answer, you can assume that you are okay to give first aid. Then, check the person's **ABCs (Airway, Breathing, Circulation)**:

- **Airway**: If the person doesn't seem to be responding, ask them out loud if they're okay and if they can open their eyes. As long as they answer, you can leave them where they are until help comes. Check their breathing, pulse, and amount of response while you wait. If the person doesn't answer, leave them where they are and open their airway, but if this can't be done where they are, gently lay them on their back and try to get it open. To do that, put one hand on the person's forehead and slightly tilt their head back while lifting the tip of their chin with two fingers. The tongue will move away from the back of the throat, but if you press on the floor of your mouth, the tongue will move up and block the airway.
  If you think the person might have hurt their spine, put your hands on either side of their head and slowly lift the angle of their jaw forward and upwards with your fingertips. This will open their airway without moving their head, so be careful not to move the neck of the person, but getting the mouth open is more important than fixing a neck injury.
- **Breathing**: To see if someone is still breathing, watch their chest move up and down, listen for breathing sounds over their mouth and nose, and feel their breath against your cheek for 10 seconds. If they're breathing regularly, put them in a side recovery position to keep their airway clear, and keep an eye on

[208] National Health Service - https://www.nhs.uk/conditions/first-aid/after-an-accident (Reviewed in March 2022)

their breathing to make sure it stays normal. To set someone at the **recovery position**:

- Kneel down next to the person who is lying on their back.
- Hold out the arm closest to you so that it is straight out from their body and the hand faces up.
- On their other arm, fold it in half so that the back of their hand rests on the closest cheek to you, and hold it in place.
- Bend the knee of the person who is the farthest away from you at a right angle with your free hand.
- Take care to turn the person over on their side by pulling on the bent knee.
- Their bent arm should hold up their head, and their straight arm will keep you from rolling them too far.
- Check to see that their bent leg is at the right angle.
- Gently tilt their head back and lift their chin to open their mouth, ensuring that nothing is blocking their airway.
- Stay with the person until help comes and keep an eye on their health.

This video from NHS will show how to set someone correctly at the recovery position:
https://youtu.be/TRQePNmR66w?si=SmQtKliscvDRB8GK

Call 911 for an ambulance if the person isn't breathing or isn't breathing regularly, and then, start CPR (next chapter).

- **Circulation**: Start chest compressions right away if the person isn't breathing properly. In the minutes after a sudden cardiac arrest (when the heart stops beating), people often breathe in and out in different ways. An irregular and rapid gasp for air is called agonal breathing. This is not the same as regular breathing, and CPR needs to be done right away. As soon as you hear that someone isn't breathing, you should call 911 for aid and start CPR.

Call: If the person answers, find out if you need to call EMS. If his/her life is in danger, do not drive to the hospital. When you go to other countries, make sure you always know the emergency numbers. 911 is used in North America, while 112 is common in the European Union and many other places around the world.

Care: First, take care of conditions that could kill you. If someone gets hurt in an accident, make sure that neither you nor the person who got hurt are in any danger. If you are, make sure everyone is safe. As much as you know and have been trained, give the care that is needed.

Choking[209]

As a person chokes, they may hold on to their chest or neck and not be able to speak, breathe, or cough.

1. Tell someone to **cough** if they are choking. You will have to help them if the blockage is very bad.
2. **Bend** them forward and **hit** them in the back up to 5 times to try to get the blockage out. Use the bottom of your hand to hit them hard on the back between the shoulder blades. When you hit them on the back, the airway is strongly vibrated and under a lot of pressure, which is usually enough to clear the blockage.

[209] British Red Cross - https://www.redcross.org.uk/first-aid/learn-first-aid/choking (Accessed in May 2024)

Watch the respective video prepared by British Red Cross:
https://youtu.be/6E9AXXRdkfE?si=xDoSz3PqFfVyrPTh

3. If they are still choking, use the **Heimlich method** to give them **abdominal thrusts**:
    - Get behind the person who is struggling to breathe.
    - Bend them forward and wrap your arms around their waist.
    - Make a fist and put it right above their belly button.
    - Rest your other hand on top of your fist and pull sharply in and up.
    - Do this move up to 5 times.

    When you do abdominal thrusts, you force air out of your lungs, which may help move the blockage. These should not be done on babies younger than 1 year old or women who are pregnant. Watch this video by WebMD to learn well this maneuver:
    https://youtu.be/xtYSTrjKonU?si=FvSd3dj99VceCFGc

4. If they are still choking call **Emergency** number.

If you're **by yourself** and choking, call 911 right away, even if you cannot speak, and then do abdominal thrusts yourself to get the object out of your throat:

- Put your fist a little above your belly.
- Use the other hand to hold your fist.
- Bend over something hard. It's okay to use a table or chair.
- Squeeze your fist in and up.

Watch this video to see the proper technique by yourself:
https://youtu.be/EunauWI4lFQ?si=gTlKEPNn_pDKjjnl

In the last years, many **devices** to stop people from choking have been made and put on the market. For lack of a power source, they work on the principle of a mechanical vacuum, and most of them use a mask that is connected to grab air from the patient's mouth and nose.
"A more detailed review of the studies demonstrated a very low certainty of evidence for its use," according to a 2020 systematic review of the effectiveness of 3 devices on the list. The review also found that "there are many weaknesses in the available data and few unbiased trials that test the effectiveness of anti-choking suction devices resulting in insufficient evidence to support or discourage their use". Practitioners

should continue to follow the guidelines made by the local resuscitation authorities.[210]

CPR/AED[211]

Heart Attack

When blood flow to part of the heart muscle is cut off, like from coronary artery disease, this is called a heart attack. These cells die because they aren't getting the oxygen and nutrients they need in the part of the heart muscle that is hurt, and this damages the heart muscle permanently. As soon as you notice the signs of a heart attack, you should get medical help right away. This can help protect the heart and even save the person's life.

Every minute counts for someone who is having a heart attack.

If you believe someone is having a heart attack, please call the emergency line right away. Believe in your gut. A lot of people who are having a heart attack wait to get help because they think they are just dealing with something small that will go away on its own, like indigestion, heartburn, a muscle strain, or the flu. There is a lot of worry about getting an ambulance and going to the emergency room for a "false alarm." There are, however, 2 hours between the first signs of a heart attack and death in most people who have one, and early improved medical care can help to lessen the damage to the heart even if the heart attack doesn't kill the person.

---

[210] Resuscitation Journal - https://www.resuscitationjournal.com/article/S0300-9572(20)30087-3/abstract (Published in August 2020)

[211] American Red Cross - https://www.redcross.org/content/dam/redcross/uncategorized/11/RTE_Textbook_Sample.pdf (Accessed in May 2024)

You should do the following if you think someone is having a heart attack:

- Call the emergency number right away. You should never try to drive someone who is having a heart attack to the hospital by yourself, because Emergency Medical Services personnel can transport the person to the hospital safely while initiating care
- Tell them to stop what they're doing and rest in a comfy place so their heart doesn't need as much oxygen. It's easier for many people having a heart attack to breathe when they're sitting down
- Loosen up any clothes that are too tight or uncomfortable
- Boost the person's confidence
- If the person has a history of heart disease and takes nitroglycerin or other prescribed medication for chest pain, offer to find the medicine and help them take it
- If the person can chew and swallow and is okay with taking aspirin, you can give them two low-dose (81 mg) aspirin pills or one regular-strength (5-grain, 325 mg) tablet
- Keep a close eye on the person's state until help arrives from Emergency Medical Services. Pay attention to any changes in how the person looks or acts
- Should you know how to do CPR and use an automatic external defibrillator (AED), you should be ready to do both if the person stops breathing

Cardiac arrest

Cardiac arrest and a heart attack are not the same thing. As you may remember, a heart attack happens when blood flow is cut off to a part of the heart muscle, and this kills that part of the heart muscle. On the other hand, cardiac arrest happens when the heart stops moving or beats too slowly to get blood to the brain and other important organs. Cardiac arrest makes the electrical signals go crazy and out of order, or they may not happen at all. In this case, the heart either stops beating or stops beating in a regular way.

The body can't stay alive for long when the heart stops beating right, and soon, there will be no more breathing, and the organs will no longer get the air they need to work. Without air, brain damage can start in 4 to 6 minutes, and after 8 to 10 minutes, the damage may be too far gone to fix. It only takes minutes for someone to die if they don't get help right away.

About 4 out of every 5 cardiac deaths in the US happen somewhere other than a hospital.

You might see someone quickly fall down when they are having a cardiac arrest. You will find that the person is not responding and is only gasping for air when you check on them. His/her heart isn't beating.

The Cardiac Chain of Survival lists 5 actions that, when done quickly one after the other, make it more likely that the person will survive cardiac arrest. You can take the first **3 actions**:

- Tell someone to **call** the emergency number right away, and someone else to look for the closest **AED (Automated External Defibrillator)**.
- Start **CardioPulmonary Resuscitation (CPR)** right away to make sure that brain and other critical organs keep getting oxygenated blood.
    1. Make sure the person is **lying** flat on their back with their face up. Before you start, quickly move the person to the floor if they are on a soft surface like a couch or bed. Get down on your knees next to them.
    2. Put your **hands in place**. Set the heel of one hand on the person's sternum, which is the bone that runs through the middle of the chest. If you feel the notch at the end of the breastbone, move your hand closer to the head of the person. You can hold your fingers together or cross them over so that they are not touching the person's chest. Place your other hand on top of the first hand.
    3. **Squeeze** the person 30 times. Set up your body so that your hands are right below your shoulders. You can then push on your chest in a straight down-and-up action, which gets the most blood moving and doesn't tire you

out as quickly. Push down at least 2 inches (5 centimeters) while keeping your arms straight. Then, let your chest return to its normal position. Do your best to push quickly and hard! Around 100 to 120 compressions per minute is what you should do. As you stretch and squeeze, count out loud to 30. Keep the down-and-up rhythm smooth and steady, and don't stop between compressions.

4. Take 2 **rescue breaths** to help the person. First, use the head-tilt/chin-lift move to open the airway. Close their nose with your finger. In order to give the first rescue breath, take a normal breath and cover the person's mouth with yours. Then, blow into their mouth. Make a seal with your breath, and then give the second saving breath. The person should feel their chest rise with each rescue breath that lasts about one second. As soon as you're done with the second set of rescue breaths, start giving compressions again. It shouldn't take more than 10 seconds to do 2 rescue breaths and then go back to compressions. You should only do 2 emergency breaths at a time.
   If the first rescue breath doesn't make the chest rise, re-drill the head to make sure the airway is open properly. Then, seal the person's nose and mouth before giving the second rescue breath. If the chest doesn't rise with the second breath, something might be in the airway. One change you should make to CPR is to open the person's mouth and look for something in it before giving rescue breaths. If you see something, take it out.

Watch this video of the American Heart Association to see how to correctly perform the CPR:
https://youtu.be/M4ACYp75mjU?si=IUHcJ8EVqwV0pLzs

Do 30 chest compressions and 2 rescue breaths every minute until you see a clear sign of life, like movement, or until an AED (Automated External Defibrillator) is ready to use and no other skilled responders are nearby to help you use it.

- Use an **AED (Automated External Defibrillator)** right away. For some people who have rapid cardiac arrest, this can fix the problem at its source. There are different kinds of AEDs, but they are all pretty easy to use and can guide the person who comes to help with either visual or audible directions. A woman who is pregnant can use an AED without getting hurt. Before using an AED, you don't have to take off the person's metal jewelry or piercings, but you should keep the pads away from any of them.
  To use an AED:
    1. **Turn on** the device. Take off or cut off the person's clothes to show their chest. Use a towel or cotton pad to dry the person's chest if it's wet.
    2. Put the **AED pads on**. Put one pad on the upper right side of the person's chest and the other on the lower left side, below the elbow, and press down hard to stick. If you need to, plug the connector wire into the AED and then follow the device's instructions. People shouldn't

touch the person while the AED is checking their heart rate, as this could lead to wrong reading.

3. Next, the AED will tell you to press the **"shock" button** if it thinks you should. As before, don't touch the person since anyone touching the person while the gadget is giving them a shock could also get a shock. After an AED shock is given (or if the AED decides that no shock is needed), start compressions right away and continue CPR. More than twice a minute, the AED will keep checking the heart rate. Pay attention to what the AED says and use it until you see a clear sign of life or until emergency medical services come. If you see a clear sign of life, stop CPR, leave the AED on and the pads on the person's chest, and keep following the AED's instructions.

Watch this video of the American Heart Association to see how to correctly use the AED:
https://youtu.be/YWyU1IRaMGs?si=QbbZfJKhbPsHEx_k

Other critical emergencies[212]

Here are some of the most common injuries that may need to be treated right away, along with tips on how to handle them.

Anaphylaxis, also called **anaphylactic shock**, is a very bad allergic reaction that can happen after eating certain foods or being stung by a bug. The bad reaction can happen very quickly, just seconds or minutes after the person comes into touch with the substance they are allergic to (allergen). When someone is in anaphylaxis shock, their tongue and throat may swell up and block their airway, making it hard for them to breathe. Check to see if the person has any medicine with them, because some people who know they have serious allergies may carry an adrenaline self-injector, which is a type of syringe that is already filled. You can help the person to take his/her medicine, or you can give it yourself if you know how. After giving the shot, keep taking care of the person until help comes.

Bleeding heavily. If you have throwaway gloves, put them on to stop the spread of infection. Make sure there isn't anything stuck in the cut.

- If there is, be careful not to press down on it. To avoid putting pressure on the object itself, press hard on both sides of it and wrap padding around it before putting on the bandage. Do not try to take it off because the object may be stopping the bleeding.
- If there is nothing stuck in the cut, put pressure on it with your gloved hand, with a clean pad or dressing if you can. Put pressure on it again and again until the blood stops. To make a strong patch, use a clean dressing or any clean, soft material. If the cut keeps bleeding through the pad, press on it until the bleeding stops. Then, put another pad on top of it and bandage it in place. Check to see if the bleeding has stopped, but don't take off the first pad or covering.

---

[212] National Health Service - https://www.nhs.uk/conditions/first-aid (Reviewed in March 2022)

If a body part has been cut off, like a finger, put it in a plastic bag or wrap it in cling film. Do not wash the limb that was cut off. Put the package in a jar of crushed ice and wrap it in soft cardboard. Keep the limb from touching the ice.

Burns and scalds:

1. Run cool water over the burn as quickly as possible for at least 20 minutes, or until the pain goes away.
2. Carefully take off any clothes or jewelry that isn't attached to the skin while the burn cools down and before it starts to swell.
3. If you cool a big burn, especially on babies, kids, or the elderly, be aware that it could lead to hypothermia. You may need to stop cooling the burn to keep the person from getting hypothermia.
4. If the burn is no longer hot, put cling film over it in a loose way. If you don't have cling film, use a clean, dry dressing or something that doesn't fluff up. If you wrap the burn too tightly, the swelling could cause more damage.
5. Don't put any lotions, creams, or sprays on the burn.

Drowning: If someone is having trouble in the water, don't go into it until it's safe to do so. Do not put yourself in danger. As soon as the person lands, you need to make sure they can breathe.

Electric shock (domestic): Break the connection between the person and the power source by turning off the electricity at the mains if someone has been shocked.
Do not touch or go near the person until you are sure that the power has been turned off if you can't get to the mains cord. In the event that the power is turned off and the person is not breathing, please call 911 for emergency medical services.

Fractures: It can be hard to tell if someone has a broken bone or joint, as opposed to a simple muscle injury, so whenever you're not sure, it's best to guess that the bone is broken. If the person is awake, keep the fracture as still as possible until you can get them to the hospital safely, since this will stop any more pain or damage. You could drive them to the hospital if the pain isn't too bad, and if possible, have someone else drive so you can take care of the person who got hurt on the trip. However, you should call 911 and do not move the person if he/she is in a lot of pain and needs strong painkillers, or has broken a leg or the back.

Do not give the hurt person anything to eat or drink because they might need anesthetic when they get to the hospital.

Poisoning: People often get poisoned by swallowing something toxic, like bleach, or by taking too much of a prescription drug. Other common reasons are eating something like wild plants and fungi.

If you swallow something poisonous, you might vomit, lose awareness, feel pain, or feel like your body is burning. The signs of alcohol poisoning can be the same.

These tips are very important: find out what the person swallowed so you can tell the paramedics or doctor; don't give them anything to eat or drink unless a doctor or nurse tells you to; don't try to make them throw up; and stay with them because their condition could get worse and they could pass out.

While you're waiting for help to arrive, if the person passes out, make sure they are breathing and do CPR if needed.

Do not use mouth-to-mouth CPR on someone whose mouth or airway is contaminated with poison.

If they are unconscious, don't leave them because they might throw up, and the puke could then get into their lungs and make them choke.

If they do vomit on their own, try to get some of it for the ambulance crew, as this could help them figure out what poisoned them.

Shock: When someone is really hurt or sick, you should watch out for signs of shock, which is when the circulatory system doesn't pump enough oxygenated blood to the body.

Most of the time, this happens after a lot of blood loss, but it can also happen after serious burns, vomiting, a heart attack, a bacterial infection, or a severe allergic reaction.
This kind of shock is different from the mental state of being shocked, which can also happen after an accident.
Pale, cold, and wet skin, sweating, fast and shallow breathing, feeling weak and dizzy, feeling sick and possibly throwing up, thirst, yawning, and sighing are all signs of shock.
As soon as possible, call 911 and ask for an ambulance. Treat any obvious injuries, lay the person down if their injuries allow it and, if possible, raise and support their legs. Keep them warm with a coat or blanket and don't give them anything to eat or drink. Give them lots of comfort and reassurance, in addition to keeping an eye on him/her. If they stop breathing, start CPR and call 911 to let them know what's going on.

To apply heat or cold?[213]

Because **cold** slows blood flow, it lessens pain and swelling, so if you have a bump, sprain, strain, pulled muscle, or severe joint pain, ice is the best thing to put on it. If the wound is less than 2 to 4 weeks old, it is called acute, and after getting hurt, it's best to put ice on it right away and keep doing so for the next 24 to 72 hours. This lowers swelling and bruises, which is important because they can hurt the flesh even more.
Ice helps the body heal, and it can still work to treat injuries for up to 2 weeks after they happen. If your symptoms last longer than a few weeks, you can try heating your muscles to help them relax.
People don't have to use ice cubes when they talk about applying ice, seeing that they can use anything cold.

Heat makes it easier for blood and nutrients to get to a part of the body, and most of the time, it works best for stiff muscles in the morning or to warm them up before activity. When you have long-term pain or

---

[213] Hospital for Special Surgery - https://www.hss.edu/article_ice-or-heat.asp (Published in September 2021)

stiffness that has gone down, heat is best. A chronic injury is one that has been going on for more than 4 weeks or one that happened a long time ago but still isn't better. If you've just hurt yourself, you should never use heat in the first few days, for the reason that putting heat on your situation can make it worse by causing more inflammation.

Wrap the pack in a small towel to help **protect your skin** whether you use heat or cold, as well as put it on the sore spot for 15 to 20 minutes several times a day.
After putting on the compress, your skin may look a little pinker whether you use heat or cold. That's normal, but don't put more ice or heat on your skin until it's back to its normal color and temperature.
If you notice any of these things after taking off the compress, you should call your doctor, since these signs show that the temperature was too extreme and could have hurt the skin: having skin that is purple-red, dark red, or a mix of red and white spots; hives; swelling; and blisters.

Drugs

Psychoactive drugs are substances that change mental processes like perception, consciousness, cognition, mood, and feelings when they are taken in. Psychoactive drugs are in a larger group of substances that can make you feel high, which also includes nicotine and booze.
Many health problems can happen if you use psychoactive drugs without a doctor's care, and these problems can even turn into drug use disorders. People with drug use disorders are more likely to get sick and die, and they can cause a lot of pain and problems in their personal, family, social, educational, occupational, or other important areas of their lives if they are not handled.

About 500,000 deaths a year around the **world** are thought to be caused by drug use, with about 350,000 deaths being men and 150,000 women.

Drug use caused more than 42 million healthy life years to be lost in 2017. That's about 1.3% of the world's disease load.[214]
It has become clear in the **Americas** that drug use is a major cause of disability and death. Moreover, in that area, the number of deaths from drug use diseases rose almost 3 times as much from 2000 to 2019. Also, this is the only region where drug use disorder is one of the top 10 causes of healthy life-years lost through early deaths and disability. In all other areas, drug use does not make the top 25.[215]

Most of the time, people **use drugs**:

- **To feel good**. Using drugs can make you feel very happy, and after this initial feeling of happiness, there are other effects that depend on the drug used. When you take drugs like cocaine, for example, you feel powerful, confident, and full of energy after the high. Opioids, like heroin, work differently, because they make you feel happy, but then they make you feel calm and satisfied.
- **To feel better**. Some people who have sadness, stress, or social anxiety start taking drugs to help them feel better. Stress can be a big reason why people start using drugs, keep using them, or go back to using them after having stopped.
- **To do better**. Some people feel like they need to increase their attention at work, in school, or in sports. This can be a reason to try drugs like cocaine or prescription stimulants.
- **Curiosity and social pressure**. Teenagers are especially at risk in this way because group pressure can be very strong. Teenage years are a time of growth and change, and having friends who use drugs is one of the things that can make someone start using drugs.

---

[214] World Health Organization - https://www.who.int/health-topics/drugs-psychoactive (Accessed in May 2024)
[215] World Health Organization - https://www.who.int/news/item/09-12-2020-who-reveals-leading-causes-of-death-and-disability-worldwide-2000-2019 (Published in December 2020)

Addiction[216]

An addiction is a long-term, relapsing problem that causes people to want and use drugs even when they know it will hurt them. It's a disorder of the brain because it changes the way reward, stress, and self-control work in parts of the brain. Many times, these changes continue even after a person stops using drugs.

When someone uses a drug for the first time, they might feel what seem like good results. Moreover, they may think they can manage how they are used. A person's life can quickly become controlled by drugs, though. As drug use goes on, other things that used to be fun become less fun, and the person needs to use drugs just to feel "normal". It's hard for them to control their urges to use drugs, even though it hurts them and those they care about. Although they may only be starting to use drugs, some people may feel like they need to take more of them or do them more often. These are the signs of being hooked.

Like many other diseases and disorders, the chance of becoming hooked to drugs is different for each person, and there is no one thing that can guarantee that someone will become addicted.

The main **risk factors** are:

- **Biological factors**: Scientists think that between 40 and 60% of a person's chance of addiction is due to their genes and the way their environment affects how those genes are expressed (this is called epigenetics). Young people and people with mental illnesses are also more likely to use drugs and become addicted than other people.
- **Family and home**. The setting at home is very important, especially when you are a child. Kids are more likely to have drug problems in the future if their parents or other older family members use drugs or too much booze as well as break the law.

---

[216] National Institute of Drug Abuse - https://nida.nih.gov/publications/drugs-brains-behavior-science-addiction/drug-misuse-addiction (Published in July 2020)

- **School and Peers**. Teenage years are a time when friends and other teens can have a bigger impact on your life. Teenagers who use drugs can get those who aren't at risk to try drugs for the first time. Kids who are having trouble in school or with their social skills may be more likely to use drugs or become hooked to them.
- **Early use**. Drug abuse can happen to anyone at any age, but studies show that people are more likely to have major problems the younger they start using drugs. This might be because drugs can damage a brain that is still growing.
- **How the drug is taken**. When you smoke or inject a drug, it makes more likely that you will become addicted to it. In these ways drugs get into the brain very quickly and give the user a strong rush of pleasure. This strong high can go away after a few minutes, though. Scientists think that this strong difference is what makes some people keep using drugs to get back to that short-lived happy state.

Therapy for drug abuse usually doesn't cure it, just like it doesn't cure most other long-term diseases like diabetes, asthma, or heart disease. On the other hand, addiction can be treated and controlled well. There is a chance that someone who is healing from an addiction will use drugs again for many years, or even their whole lives. Research has shown that most people have the best chance of success when they use both medication and behavioral therapy to help their addiction. Treatment plans that are customized to each person's drug use habits and any medical, mental, or social issues that may be present can help them stay sober.

An article in The Lancet **compared 20 drugs** based on their harm and dependence risk. They used a scale from 0 to 3 for physical dependence, psychological dependence, and pleasure to arrive at a mean score for reliance.

Selected results can be seen in the following chart.[217]

Drug	Mean	Pleasure	Psychological dependence	Physical dependence
Heroin/Morphine	3.00	3.0	3.0	3.0
Cocaine	2.39	3.0	2.8	1.3
Tobacco	2.21	2.3	2.6	1.8
Barbiturates	2.01	2.0	2.2	1.8
Alcohol	1.93	2.3	1.9	1.6
Benzodiazepines	1.83	1.7	2.1	1.8
Amphetamine	1.67	2.0	1.9	1.1
Cannabis	1.51	1.9	1.7	0.8
Ecstasy	1.13	1.5	1.2	0.7

Opioid overdose[218]

Almost 80% of drug-related deaths around the world are caused by opioids, and about 25% of those deaths are due to overdose. In 2021, around 60 million people used opioids at least once.

The word "opioids" refers to chemicals that come from the **poppy plant** (papaver somniferum) as well as semisynthetic and synthetic chemicals that have similar effects and can connect with opioid receptors in the brain.

Opioids can make people feel good after taking them, which is one of the main reasons why people use them for reasons other than medical ones. Heroin, morphine, codeine, fentanyl, methadone, tramadol, and other drugs like these are opioids.

---

[217] The Lancet - https://www.thelancet.com/journals/lancet/article/PIIS0140-6736(07)60464-4/fulltext (Published in March 2007)

[218] World Health Organization - https://www.who.int/news-room/fact-sheets/detail/opioid-overdose (Published in August 2023)

Because of **how they work** in the body, opioids can make it hard to breathe, and an overdose can kill you.
Males, older people, and people with low incomes are at higher risk.
A lot of things can make you more likely to overdose on opioids, and some of these are: having an opioid use disorder; injecting opioids; starting to use opioids again after a long break; using prescription opioids without a doctor's supervision; taking more opioids than prescribed; using opioids with alcohol or other drugs that make it hard to breathe, like benzodiazepines, barbiturates, anesthetics, or some painkillers; and having another medical condition at the same time, like HIV, liver or lung diseases, or mental issues.

There are effective ways to **treat** opioid dependence that can lower the chance of overdose, but less than 10% of people who need it are getting it.

Cocaine[219]

In 2015, 1.9 million people aged 12 and up in the **US** used cocaine in the past month. It was determined that about 900,000 of them had a disorder that could be diagnosed and had major negative affects because of their cocaine use in the past year. Overdoses and deaths from cocaine use went up by 42% in 2014.

Cocaine gives users a short-lived high that makes them more alert, talkative, and energized. This high can be followed by restlessness, anger, and fear. Cocaine is very **addictive** and can make you more likely to experience mental illnesses like psychosis, confusion, and anxiety.
Several times, people who use cocaine don't eat or sleep at healthy times, they might have a faster heartbeat, muscle twitches, and convulsions. Snorting cocaine can also damage nose tissue in a way that can't be fixed.

---

[219] Substance Abuse and Mental Health Services Administration - https://store.samhsa.gov/sites/default/files/d7/priv/pep18-01.pdf (Revised in 2018)

Drug **abuse** can lead to seizures, strokes, comas, and heart attacks.
It is very dangerous to mix cocaine with other drugs, and it is especially dangerous with alcohol because when they mix, they make cocaethylene, a drug that is much more dangerous than either cocaine or alcohol by itself.

Quitting smoking

In the United States, smoking is the **main reason people die too soon and could have been avoided**. About 480,000 people die too soon every year in the United States because they smoke cigarettes or are exposed to tobacco smoke. About 39% of these early deaths are caused by heart disease or stroke, 36% by cancer, and 24% by lung disease. People who smoke have about 3 times higher death rates than people who have never smoked. Almost every organ system in the body is hurt by smoking, which is bad for general health.
Women who smoke have a harder time getting pregnant: miscarriages, ectopic pregnancies, babies born too early and with an abnormally low birth weight, and babies born with cleft lip and cleft palate are more likely to happen to pregnant women who smoke.
The longer a person smokes, the more likely is that smoking will hurt them or even cause them to die younger. But smokers of any age can greatly lower their risk of getting sick, including cancer, by giving up the habit.
Nicotine use can also hurt the growing brain of a teen until about age 25. Teenagers who use nicotine can hurt the parts of their brain that manage mood, learning, attention, and impulses. Also, using tobacco as a teen may make it more likely that you will become addicted to other drugs in the future.
You can't smoke at any level. If you smoke even one cigarette a day for your whole life, you could get lung, bladder, or liver cancer and die too soon.

Third-party smoke, which is also known as passive smoking, is made up of "mainstream" smoke (the smoke a user breathes out) and "side stream" smoke (the smoke a tobacco product burns). Around 7,300 adult nonsmokers die each year in the United States from lung cancer after being exposed to secondhand smoke. The U.S. Surgeon General says that living with a smoker raises the risk of lung cancer in people who don't smoke by 20% to 30%.[220]

What happens **when you quit**?[221]

- After 20 minutes: check your heart rate, it should return to normal.
- After 8 hours: your oxygen levels will be back to normal, and the harmful amount of carbon monoxide in your blood will have dropped by half.
- After 48 hours: there is no more carbon dioxide. Your lungs are getting rid of gunk, and you can taste and smell better.
- After 72 hours: if you feel like it's easier to breathe, that's because your lung tubes have begun to loosen up. You will also have more energy.
- After 2 to 12 weeks: your circulation will be better, letting more blood flow to your heart and muscles.
- After 3 to 9 months: your coughs, wheezing, and breathing problems will get better as your lung function rises by up to 10%.
- After 1 year: Great news! Your chance of having a heart attack will be half of what it is for someone who smokes.
- After 10 years: more good news! Your chance of dying from lung cancer will be half of what it is for someone who smokes.

It's not easy to stop smoking because it's so addictive, and this is for the **nicotine** in them. Nicotine is what keeps people smoking even when they really want to quit, but it's the thousands of chemicals in tobacco

---

[220] National Cancer Institute - https://www.cancer.gov/about-cancer/causes-prevention/risk/tobacco/cessation-fact-sheet (Reviewed in December 2017)
[221] National Health Service - https://www.nhs.uk/better-health/quit-smoking (Accessed in May 2024)

that make it so dangerous. People who smoke tobacco are more likely to get lung illnesses like chronic obstructive pulmonary disease (COPD) and cancer because of this dangerous mix of chemicals, not nicotine. Different amounts of nicotine in tobacco goods are bad for adults' health in different ways.[222]

- **Combustible products**, or products that burn tobacco, are the most dangerous. A flammable product is a cigarette, which has more than 7,000 chemicals in it. Studies have shown that cigar smoke has higher amounts of harmful chemicals than cigarette smoke, but people don't usually breathe in cigar smoke like they do cigarette smoke. Oral, larynx, stomach, pancreas, and lung cancer can be caused by smoking cigars. Also, people who smoke cigars every day, especially those who inhale, have a higher chance of getting heart disease and other lung diseases. Concerning hookah (also known as waterpipe, shisha, and narghile), some people believe that smoking it is less harmful and addictive than smoking cigarettes. However, studies have shown that hookah smoke is at least as harmful as cigarette smoke.
- **Noncombustible products**, such as Heated Tobacco Products – HTP (IQOS is one example), e-cigarettes, and smokeless tobacco. There are a lot of different kinds of heats tobacco products, which are sometimes sold as "heat-not-burn" goods. They're not the same as e-cigarettes because HTPs heat real tobacco leaves, while e-cigarettes heat liquids that usually have nicotine from tobacco along with flavorings and other things. It is usually thought that the emissions from HTPs have fewer harmful chemicals than cigarette smoke, but that doesn't mean heated tobacco is safe. We are still learning about the short- and long-term health effects of HTPs because they are still new. According to research, heated tobacco products and the smoke they make

---

[222] Food and Drug Administration - https://www.fda.gov/tobacco-products/health-effects-tobacco-use/nicotine-why-tobacco-products-are-addictive (Published in June 2022)

have many of the same harmful chemicals as normal cigarettes, and they also have even some harmful chemicals that aren't in regular cigarettes. More study is needed to find out if adult smokers who move to heated tobacco products might lower their chances of getting a disease related to smoking. Studies show that most people who use HTPs still smoke cigarettes. Multiple tobacco products use is linked to a higher chance of nicotine dependence and other health problems. The FDA has only allowed one HTP system to be sold as modified risk tobacco products: this is IQOS and 3 of its Heatstick items that contain tobacco. This was the first time that "exposure modification" orders were given for tobacco goods. People who smoke regular cigarettes and then switch to IQOS may be told that they are less likely to be exposed to chemicals that are bad for them.[223]

As of now, no e-cigarette has been approved as a way to help people quit smoking or been given permission to make a modified risk claim, and more study is needed to fully understand the risks and benefits these products may have for adults who smoke.

Oral, spit, dip, chew, snus, dissolvable, and snuff tobacco are all types of smokeless tobacco. Oral (mouth, tongue, cheek, and gum), esophageal, and pancreatic cancers are all caused by smokeless tobacco, moreover it may also cause gum and heart disease.

- The safest are **Nicotine Replacement Treatments (NRTs).** NRT products are safe and work well to help adults stop smoking, and they do this by sending small amounts of nicotine to the brain without the harmful chemicals that are in cigarette smoke. NRTs like nicotine skin patches, gum, and lozenges, can help you stop by easing nicotine withdrawal symptoms and cravings.

[223] Centers for Disease Control and Prevention - https://www.cdc.gov/tobacco/basic_information/heated-tobacco-products/index.html (Reviewed in November 2023)

People often try to **quit smoking** on their own, but getting help is much more likely to help them stay smoke-free. There are many ways to get help, so find a mix that works for you:[224, 225]

- **Vaping** to quit smoking: Vapes are electric gadgets that let you breathe in nicotine as a vapor instead of smoke. This is done by heating an e-liquid solution that usually has nicotine, flavorings, propylene glycol, and veggie glycerin in it. There are different nicotine levels in e-liquids, so you can decide how much nicotine you need to help with cravings and other withdrawal symptoms, like being irritable and sad. Nicotine isn't really dangerous, and it's been used safely in drugs to help people quit smoking for a long time, so vaping nicotine is a lot less dangerous than smoking. It also helps people quit smoking better than anything else. Vaping isn't totally safe, and we only suggest it to adult smokers who want to help themselves quit and stay quit. Vaping hasn't been around long enough for us to know what risks come with using it for a long time.
- Stop smoking **aids**: therapies that help people stop smoking really help with nicotine cravings and other withdrawal symptoms. They also make it more likely that you will be able to quit, especially if you get help from a local group that helps people stop smoking. Ask your health care provider what they think. A lot of people don't take their medicines properly, for long enough, or at all. Make sure to follow the advice and use other tools to help you quit along with the medicine. If you get professional help, you're 3 times more likely to quit for good.
- Pay attention to what **motivates** you. It's normal for motivation to rise and fall, therefore what can you do to boost your motivation when you feel beaten or down?

---

[224] National Health Service - https://www.nhs.uk/better-health/quit-smoking (Accessed in May 2024)

[225] American Lung Association - https://www.lung.org/quit-smoking/i-want-to-quit/top-tips-for-quitting-smoking (Updated in May 2023)

- Boost your **confidence**. It is important to have faith that your try will work! What can you do to feel surer of yourself? You can feel more confident when you set and reach a number of small goals, when you picture yourself succeeding, and when you know you have everything you need to handle any situation.
- Dealing with **stress** is very important. A lot of smokers do it to deal with worry, anxiety, and bad feelings, so it can be hard and take a lot of practice to be ready with other ways to deal with these thoughts. How do your friends who don't smoke deal with stress?
- It's **never too late** to quit. Of course, giving up smoking as soon as possible is ideal, but you can do it at any age and make your life better. Plus, you won't have to go outside in the cold to smoke, as well as it will save you money.
- Pick up **lessons** from the past. Most smokers have tried to quit before, and sometimes the thought of those failed attempts makes them give up. But these events teach us a lot about what to do next time and what not to do! These things you've done are steps toward future success. This time, think about what worked, what didn't, and what you could do better.
- You don't have to quit **by yourself**. It will be easier to quit if you tell your friends and family about it and ask them to help you.
- **Anyone** can quit. Friends who smoke may even join you in your efforts. There are many ways to try to quit because everyone is different. Discover the best mix of tools, medicines, and help for you! Above all, don't give up.

Alcohol misuse[226]

Having too much alcohol can **lead to** more than 200 diseases, injuries, and other health problems. People who drink alcohol are more likely to have health problems, such as mental and behavioral issues, including alcohol dependence, as well as major noncommunicable diseases like heart disease, liver cirrhosis, and some types of cancer.
Every year, 3 million people die around the world because they drink too much. This is equal to 5.3% of all deaths. Alcohol use leads to death and injury pretty early in life, and more specifically 13% of all deaths in people ages 20 to 39 are caused by drinking.[227]

Adults should not drink more than **14 units of alcohol a week** to keep low the health risks from drinking.
A unit of alcohol is 8 grams or 10 milliliters of pure alcohol, and this is equal to half a pint of low- to moderate-strength beer or cider (ABV Alcohol By Volume 3.6%) or one small shot measure (25ml) of spirits (ABV 40%). About 1.5 units of alcohol are in a small glass (125ml) of wine (ABV 12%).
If you drink up to 14 units a week, it's best to do it over at least 3 days.

The **short-term risks** of alcohol misuse include:

- **Accidents** and injuries that need medical care, like a head injury. A lot of the injuries that are linked to drinking alcohol are caused on purpose or by accident, like those that happen in car accidents, fights, and suicide. People in younger age groups are more likely to die from accidents caused by alcohol.
- **Unprotected sex**, which could result in an unwanted pregnancy or an STD
- **Alcohol poisoning**: this can make you throw up, have seizures, and lose consciousness.

---

[226] National Health Service - https://www.nhs.uk/conditions/alcohol-misuse (Reviewed in October 2022)
[227] World Health Organization - https://www.who.int/news-room/fact-sheets/detail/alcohol (Published in May 2022)

If you drink too much alcohol on a regular basis, in the **long term** you're more likely to get heart disease, stroke, liver disease, cancer (liver, bowel, mouth, and breast), pancreatitis, and brain damage that can make it hard to think and remember things. Long-term alcohol abuse can cause major health problems and can also cause social problems for some people, like losing their jobs, getting divorced, abuse at home, or not having a place to live.

It's called dependent drinking (also called **alcoholism**) when someone can't stop drinking and wants to drink too much.
If you or someone else is worried about drinking, a good first step is to see a doctor, who will be able to talk about the treatments and services that are offered.

Hangover

A hangover refers to a set of symptoms that occur as a consequence of drinking too much, and it can vary from person to person. A hangover is mostly caused by alcohol, but other parts of alcoholic drinks may also cause headache symptoms or make them worse. **Sulfites** are chemicals that are used to keep wine from going bad, and some people who are sensitive to them may get a headache after drinking wine.

Many people on Facebook have shared the idea that the word "hangover" comes from something that British sailors did during the rule of Queen Victoria: they bought "access to hang over a rope" after a night of heavy drinking. But this claim is not true. The idea behind the word dates back to 1894 and means "a thing or person remaining or **left over**".[228]

[228] Oxford English Dictionary - https://www.oed.com/search/dictionary/?scope=HistoricalThesaurus&q=hangover (Accessed in May 2024)

Hangovers can be caused by a number of things:[229]

- Mild **dehydration:** alcohol stops the brain from releasing vasopressin, a hormone that tells the kidneys to hold on to water, which means that drinking booze makes you pee more and lose more fluids. It's possible that mild dehydration makes hangover symptoms like thirst, tiredness, and headaches worse.
- **Sleep** problems: a lot of people fall asleep faster after drinking, but their sleep is broken up, and they wake up earlier. This makes people tired and makes them less productive.
- Irritation of the **intestines**: alcohol directly irritates the stomach walls and makes it produce more acid. This could lead to nausea and give you stomach pain.
- **Inflammation**: alcohol increases inflammation in the body. Inflammation contributes to the malaise that people feel when they are sick, so it may play a role in hangover symptoms as well.
- **Acetaldehyde** exposure: the liver is the main organ that breaks down alcohol through acetaldehyde, a toxic byproduct that doesn't last long. However, this toxin can cause inflammation in the liver, pancreas, brain, gastrointestinal tract, and other organs.
- Mini withdrawal: people who drink may feel calmer, more relaxed, or even euphoric, but their brains quickly get used to these good effects as they try to keep things in balance. Because of this, people can feel more antsy and tense after drinking than they did before.

Of course, the best solution to do is to not drink any booze, but if you do drink, here are some easy **ways to feel better** afterward:[230]

---

[229] National Institute on Alcohol Abuse and Alcoholism - https://www.niaaa.nih.gov/publications/brochures-and-fact-sheets/hangovers (Updated in March 2021)

- Drinking **fluids**. You may be even more dehydrated if you have diarrhea, sweat a lot, or throw up because of your hangover. It might be hard to drink anything when you have nausea, but even a few sips of water might help your hangover.
- Getting some **carbs**. Since drinking may lower blood sugar, some of the tiredness and headaches that come with hangovers could be caused by the brain not getting enough of its main fuel. A lot of people also forget to eat when they drink, which makes their blood sugar even lower. A breakfast of toast and juice can help bring levels back to normal.
- Staying away from **darker drinks**. In tests, it was found that clear liquors like vodka and gin are less likely to give people hangovers than dark liquors like whiskey, red wine, and tequila. Most alcoholic drinks contain ethanol as their main form of alcohol, but darker liquors also contain congeners, which are chemically similar compounds like methanol. Both ethanol and methanol are broken down by the same enzymes, however, methanol molecules are more dangerous and may make your hangover worse.
- Taking **painkillers**. Other nonsteroidal anti-inflammatory drugs (NSAIDs), like aspirin and ibuprofen, may help with the headache and general pain, but on the other hand, they might irritate a stomach that is already upset by drinking. If you've been drinking booze, don't take acetaminophen (Tylenol), since it may accentuate acetaminophen's toxic effect on the liver.
- **Caffeine**. Caffeine might not be able to cure hangovers in a special way, but as a stimulant, it might help with feeling sleepy. But it's important to remember that you should never mix caffeine and alcohol because caffeine can hide the depressant effect of alcohol, making you feel more alert than you would normally.

---

[230] Harvard Health Publishing - https://www.health.harvard.edu/staying-healthy/7-steps-to-cure-your-hangover-and-ginkgo-biloba-whats-the-verdict (Published in May 2023)

- Getting **iron** and **B vitamins**. A study in The Journal of Clinical Medicine looked at the meals for 24 hours before and after people drank too much. They did find that people whose food and drinks had higher amounts of zinc and B vitamins had milder hangovers.
- **Hair of the dog**. People who drink to get over a hangover are sometimes said to be "taking the hair of the dog". People believe that hangovers are a form of alcohol withdrawals, and that having one or two drinks will help with it. But the dog's hair just keeps the loop going, so you can't get better from it.

Healthcare system and society

"Wherever the art of medicine is loved, there is also a love of Humanity"
Hippocrates (Greek physician, circa 400 BC)

Checkups[231]

Some people check in with their doctor once a year to make sure everything is fine, while some people think they don't need to go that often. At the end of the day, it depends on your age, health, and factors that put you at risk for certain problems.
Your doctor will want to know about your health and how you live, then they will likely take your vital signs and listen to your heart and lungs.
You should still get these **checks** and tests under the radar, though:

- **BMI (Body Mass Index)**: keeping it at a healthy level can help keep you from getting heart disease, type 2 diabetes, and some types of cancer.
- **Blood pressure:** heart disease and stroke are more likely to happen if it's too high. After age 18, you should have your blood pressure checked at least every 2 years, and you might need to take it more often if it's high. Talk to your doctor about how often you should take it.
- **Cholesterol**: having too much cholesterol can cause heart disease and stroke. If you are over 20, you should get your cholesterol checked every 4 to 6 years. It's possible that your doctor will tell you to get it checked more often if you are an older adult, a male, overweight, or if someone in your family has had heart disease, diabetes, or high cholesterol.
- **Blood sugar**: this is a way to find out if you have diabetes or are at risk of getting it. The test is easy and tells you how much sugar (also called glucose) is in your blood. Once you turn 45, you should start getting regular tests. If you are overweight, have high cholesterol or blood pressure, or have had gestational diabetes, your doctor may tell you to get it done sooner.
- **Skin**: look at your scars, moles, and other skin marks to see if they have changed. An expert says that you should check your own skin every month, because skin cancers can almost always

[231] WebMD - https://www.webmd.com/a-to-z-guides/ss/slideshow-checkups-needed (Reviewed in January 2022)

be cured if they are found and handled quickly. If you or someone in your family has had skin cancer, you should have your skin checked by a doctor regularly.

- **Bones density**: as you age, your bones get lighter and thinner, and over time, which can make your bones very weak and more likely to break, known as osteoporosis. For women aged 65 and up and men aged 70 and up, you should get your bone density checked. There are things that can be done if your doctor finds that your bones are weakening. If you have broken a bone in the past, taken steroids for a long time, have rheumatoid arthritis, weigh less than 127 pounds (58 kilograms), or have a parent who broke their hip after a minor accident, your doctor may want you to get this test sooner.
- **Teeth**: you might need to go to the dentist once or twice a year. Your oral health and what you need to do to keep your mouth and smile healthy will determine it.
- **Cancers**
    - **Breasts**: they will be checked for changes with this X-ray test as for a mammogram. Once you turn 40, talk to your doctor about it. They might tell you to wait until you're 50, or they might tell you to get your first one right away. After the first one, you'll get one every year or 2.
    - **Colorectal**: tests look for blood or growths of tissue called polyps in the colon or rectum to see if there is cancer there. When you turn 45, you should start getting these tests even if you don't have a high risk of getting this cancer.
    - **Cervical**: for this, there are a couple of tasks to perform. A pap test checks your cervix to see if there are any changes that could turn into cancer, then your doctor will open your vagina with a tool called a speculum and take some cells to look at. With this sample, it will be checked for HPV and for a virus that can bring about the changes in cells that can lead to cervical cancer. From about age 21,

talk to your doctor about what's best for you, you might only get one test or both.

- **Prostate**: most men will want to talk to their doctor about this around age 50. Men who are African American or who have a history of prostate cancer in their family may need to it between the ages of 40 and 45. A PSA blood test is most often used, or a rectal check might be given to you instead. What's best for you will be told by your doctor.

Advice about self-care

Doctors used to give medicines for conditions that either get better on their own (like a sore throat or a cold) or are easy to treat with safe, mild treatments. In the past, these medicines would not have been easy to get, but these days, a lot more drugs can be bought **Over-The-Counter (OTC)**, which means you can get them at any time from a pharmacy.

This chapter's main goal is not to promote these drugs, but to teach people how to use them properly.

Remember to look for the statement that lists the tamper-evident features before you buy the product and every time you use it. More does not always mean better when it comes to drugs, so you should never take over-the-counter medicines for longer or in bigger doses than what the label says. If your symptoms don't go away, it's clear that you need to see a doctor. Every time you buy something, make sure you read the label. Even if 2 or more drugs are from the same brand family, that doesn't mean they treat the same conditions or have the same ingredients. If you read the warning and are still not sure, talk to a doctor, nurse, or pharmacist.

What are the **most common** OTC drugs?[232]

- **Paracetamol**, a **pain killer**: paracetamol stops pain and fevers. Children and adults can take it as tablets, while babies and young children can take it as a drink, like Calpol. If you have little kids, paracetamol is probably the most important medicine to always have on hand. Normal amounts of paracetamol are safe, but taking too much can be dangerous, consequently it is very important to make sure to get the right amount. It is usually safe to drink a small amount of booze while taking paracetamol, but if you already have some health problems, like liver problems, it might not be a good idea to drink alcohol while taking paracetamol. It doesn't matter if you haven't eaten because paracetamol doesn't hurt the walls of the stomach.
- **Anti-inflammatory** drugs, like aspirin or ibuprofen, are pain killers that also reduce inflammation. They can help with sprains and aches in the muscles, and they can also be used to ease period pain, or to bring down fevers, just like paracetamol. Doses change based on age. You can also get anti-inflammatory as a gel or foam, so they can be rubbed right into the sore spot. Ibuprofen and paracetamol do not help the body in the same way: most of the time, paracetamol works best for pain, like headaches and stomachaches; if you have toothaches, back pain or period pain, ibuprofen might work better. It is best to take NSAIDs (Non-Steroidal Anti-Inflammatory Drugs) with food or a glass of milk because they can irritate the lining of the gut.
- **Antihistamines**, such as Cetirizine, chlorpheniramine, or fexofenadine: these help with hives (urticaria), itching, coughing, watery eyes, and runny nose that come with hay fever and other allergies. The pain and swelling from wasp or bee stings can also be eased with them. Some antihistamines, like chlorphenamine, may make you sleepy, so these might help if you have an itchy disease like eczema or chickenpox and want to

[232] MyHSN - https://www.myhsn.co.uk/top-tip/what-are-the-most-important-otc-tablets-to-keep-at-home (Accessed in May 2024)

take them before bed. From the other side, cetirizine is one type that makes you less sleepy and is better during the day. You can also buy antihistamine as a cream that you can put on stings and bites.

- **Antacids**, such as Gaviscon, sodium bicarbonate, magnesium trisilicate, aluminum, or magnesium hydroxide, can help with heartburn and indigestion. They work by making the stomach's acid less strong. In case you have to take antacids often, you should talk to your doctor about this.
- **Hydrocortisone steroid cream**: steroids lessen inflammation. You can get hydrocortisone at the pharmacy to treat eczema, dermatitis, and bug stings. It is important to remember that you should not put hydrocortisone cream on your face unless your doctor tells you to.
- **Antibiotic cream**, as bacitracin ointment, is a good thing to have on hand. Small cuts, scrapes, and bites are less likely to get infected if you use this on them.
- **Mouth ulcer gel** (bonjela): if someone in your family gets mouth sores or ulcers often, you should keep something on hand to help.
- Creams with clotrimazole, ketoconazole, miconazole, or terbinafine are **antifungal drugs** that are used to treat fungal diseases on the skin, hair, nails, and genitalia. If you have ringworm, athlete's foot, oral thrush, or fungal nappy rash, these medicines can help.
- Medicines for **diarrhea** and **constipation** (loperamide and senna): talk to your doctor if you have diarrhea or constipation for more than 3 weeks.

Even though they are usually mild and don't happen very often, **interactions** between over-the-counter drugs can cause unwanted effects or make meds less effective. When you take both prescription and over-the-counter drugs at the same time, it's even more important to know about drug combinations.

Some common over-the-counter (OTC) chemicals can interact with the following drugs:

- Don't drink alcohol if you are on antihistamines, dextromethorphan-containing cough or cold medicines, or drugs that treat sleeplessness.
- If you are already taking sedatives or tranquilizers, don't take drugs that help you sleep.
- If you have diabetes, gout, or are taking a prescription blood thinner, talk to your doctor before taking any goods that contain aspirin.
- If you have stomach pain, sickness, or vomiting, don't take laxatives.
- If you are taking a prescription drug for depression or high blood pressure, or if you have heart or thyroid disease, diabetes, or problems with your prostate, don't use a nasal decongestant unless your doctor tells you to.

This list isn't all of them, so check out the label! As new information comes in, drug labels can change, that's why you should read the label every time you take a medicine.

Always keep medicines in a cool, dry place, or follow the directions on the container. Once a year, make sure you go through your medicine cabinet, and medicines that have passed their expiration date should be thrown away. Then keep all drugs in their original containers so that no one takes the wrong one.

Drugs can be passed from a pregnant woman to her baby, and what is safe for the woman may be too much for the baby still in the womb. Even though most drugs are found in very small amounts in breast milk and won't hurt the baby, mothers who are breastfeeding should still be careful, so before taking any drugs, you should always talk to your doctor if you are pregnant or breastfeeding.

Don't guess the dose based on the child's size; kids aren't just little people.

Most over-the-counter medicines come in Tamper-Evident Packaging (TEP), which helps keep thieves from tampering with the goods, because with TEP, there is clear proof if the package has been tampered with.[233]

Generic medicines work the same as more expensive brand-name medicines, even if the pills you get at the drugstore counter look a little different. The active chemicals are the same, and the quality standards for making and packing them must be met.
The biggest difference between generic and brand-name drugs is the price, and generic manufacturers compete directly on price, which means that prices for customers are lower. Americans have saved $2.2 trillion in the last 10 years thanks to generic drugs.[234]

Prescription drugs abuse

This chapter takes a quick look at some prescription drugs that can have adverse effects on your health, like addiction, if they are used in ways or by people who aren't supposed to or as directed.
Most drug abuse happens with 3 types of drugs:[235]

- **Opioids — for pain relief**. One of the most interesting things about these drugs is how quickly some people become dependent on them. Opiates and opioids are drugs like Heroin, Codeine, Fentanyl, Hydrocodone, Morphine, Methadone, Oxycodone, and Pethidine. All of these opioids can be given by doctors, except for heroin, which is a drug that can't be bought on the street. Opiates work well for short-term pain relief, but most doctors agree that they shouldn't be used to treat chronic or long-term pain.

---

[233] Food and Drug Administration - https://www.fda.gov/drugs/choosing-right-over-counter-medicine-otcs/over-counter-medicines-whats-right-you (Published in March 2013)
[234] Association for Accessible Medicines - https://accessiblemeds.org/resources/blog/whats-difference-between-generics-and-brand-name-drugs (Accessed in May 2024)
[235] UK Addiction Treatment Centres - https://www.ukat.co.uk/addiction/drug/prescription (Accessed in May 2024)

- **Sedatives or tranquilizers** — barbiturates and benzodiazepines, prescribed for anxiety or sleep problems. 12 million prescriptions are written each year for benzodiazepines, which are a big group of drugs. In the UK, 1.5 million people are addicted to benzodiazepines because they abuse prescription drugs like Xanax, Valium, Klonopin, Ativan, and Ambien. Benzodiazepine abuse mostly happens when you self-medicate. Most of the time, this is caused by deeper problems that haven't been dealt with, like sorrow, mental health issues, trauma, or worries about money.

  Z-drugs, which are newer sleeping pills, work in a similar way. However, some people think they are less addictive, which is not true. Zolpidem and Zopiclone are 2 of these.

  For many reasons, the abuse of sleeping pills is getting worse all the time. To begin, more people than ever are getting prescriptions for sleeping pills; in addition to being over-prescribed, sleeping pills are also quite easy to get online, so this means that people whose prescriptions have run out as well as people who want to abuse sleeping pills for fun can easily get them. During the pandemic, more and more people with anxiety and insomnia turned to sleeping pills that they got secretly to deal with their problems.
- **Stimulants**—prescribed for attention-deficit hyperactivity disorder (ADHD), the sleep disorder narcolepsy, or obesity.

In 2010, approximately 16 million Americans reported using a prescription drug for nonmedical reasons in the past year; 7 million in the past month (5.1 with pain relievers, 2.6 with sedatives or tranquilizers 1.1. with stimulants).[236]

These are 5 **things to know** about prescription drug addiction:

---

[236] National Institute on Drug Abuse - https://nida.nih.gov/sites/default/files/rx_drugs_placemat_508c_10052011.pdf (Revised in October 2011)

- Being hooked on prescription drugs can be just as dangerous as being hooked on illegal drugs.
- Not all pharmaceutical drugs are dangerous: if you take your prescription drugs at the right times and in the right amounts, you are much less likely to become addicted to them.
- It may be easy for people to lie or hide the fact that they are addicted to prescription drugs: prescription drugs are not illegal, so they are easier to get and follow the law.
- Some people may have a tough time understanding drug addiction to prescription drugs: some people find it hard to understand prescription drug addiction because they have been taught stereotypical ideas about drug addiction.
- You can stop being addicted, so get help!

Complementary and Alternative Medicine[237]

Complementary and Alternative Medicine, or **CAM**, is a type of treatment that is not part of standard medicine, and no one can really agree on a single **definition** of CAM.

The US National Center for Complementary and Integrative Health (NCCIH) uses this distinction:

- When a non-mainstream practice is used together with conventional medicine, it's considered **complementary**.
- When a non-mainstream practice is used instead of conventional medicine, it's considered **alternative**.

The main idea behind some CAM treatments and the data they use are not accepted by most independent scientists. Some have been shown to help with a few specific health problems, and as an example, there is proof that chiropractic care can help with lower back pain.
The placebo effect is what might happen when someone uses any kind of health care and feels better afterward.

---

[237] National Health System - https://www.nhs.uk/conditions/complementary-and-alternative-medicine (Reviewed in March 2022)

Homeopathy, acupuncture, chiropractic care, and herbal treatments are all examples of CAM.

Homeopathy

Homeopathy is a way of treating illness that was created in Germany more than 200 years ago, and 2 unconventional **ideas** form the basis of it:

- **Like cures like** is the idea that a substance that makes healthy people have similar symptoms can fix a disease.
- **Law of minimum dose**: the idea that a medicine works better when taken in smaller amounts. A lot of homeopathic medicines are watered down so much that they don't contain even any molecules of the original material.

Plants are used to make homeopathic medicines. Homeopathy has a different way of figuring out what's wrong with a person and how to treat them, additionally it also sees different patterns in signs and symptoms than traditional medicine does.

The 2012 National Health Interview Survey asked a lot of questions about how Americans use complementary and alternative health approaches. It found that about 5 million people and 1 million children used homeopathy in the previous year.

A study on homeopathy from the House of Commons Science and Technology Committee in 2010 said that homeopathic treatments **don't work** any better than placebos.

The National Health and Medical Research Council of Australia's government looked at all the data and found in 2015 that there is no solid proof that homeopathy can help with any health problem. It is important to remember that the studies that were used in this assessment of evidence had to meet a lot of strict requirements. For example, they had to have a sample size of more than 150 people and get the highest grade for methodological quality, among other things. In total, 57 systematic reviews with 176 separate works were looked at for this evaluation.[238]

In 2017, the National Health System in England said it would no longer pay for homeopathy on the NHS because there wasn't enough proof that it worked to make the cost worth it. In 2018, the High Court agreed with this.[239]

Under the Federal Food, Drug, and Cosmetic Act in the US, homeopathic products must follow the same rules as other drug products when it comes to approval, adulteration, and misbranding, consequently the FDA has not yet cleared any homeopathic products.

FDA released a final guidance in December 2022, called "Homeopathic Drug Products", which explains how the agency will decide which homeopathic products pose the most risk to patients and how they will be regulated. Homeopathic goods labels usually say that they are highly diluted, but some of them have been found to still have measurable amounts of active ingredients, which means they could do a lot of harm to patients.[240]

Homeopathy is a touchy subject, and in conclusion some of the most important ideas in the theory of homeopathy don't fit with basic science ideas as we know them.

Acupuncture

Acupuncture is a technique that comes from traditional Chinese medicine. In some parts of the body, fine needles are inserted to treat or avoid problems, and it works by activating nerves in the muscles and under the skin.

This makes the body produce natural chemicals, like endorphins, which relieve pain. It's likely that these naturally occurring chemicals are what make acupuncture relaxing and healing.

---

[238] National Center For Complementary and Alternative Medicine - https://www.nccih.nih.gov/health/homeopathy (Updated in April 2021)

[239] National Health System - https://www.nhs.uk/conditions/homeopathy (Reviewed in April 2021)

[240] Food and Drug Administration - https://www.fda.gov/drugs/information-drug-class/homeopathic-products (Published in May 2023)

Most of the time, a course of acupuncture is suggested because you may not see results until after a few sessions.
If you decide to get acupuncture, you should make sure that the person doing it is either a licensed healthcare worker (like a doctor, nurse, or physiotherapist) or a member of a national acupuncture organization.
Acupuncture is usually very safe when done by a trained professional.[241]

Acupuncture has its **roots** in the idea that the body has meridians, which are energy pathways that carry "life force" through it. Qi (pronounced "chee"). Traditional acupuncture practitioners think that sickness can happen when Qi doesn't move freely through the body, and they also think that acupuncture can get the flow of Qi going again, which will make them healthy again.

Researchers have found that acupuncture may **help** with a number of types of pain, such as back or neck pain, knee pain from osteoarthritis, and pain after surgery. It may also help ease the pain in the joints that comes from taking aromatase inhibitors, which are drugs that people with breast cancer take. In addition to being looked at for pain, acupuncture has been looked at for at least 50 other health issues. There is some proof that acupuncture may help with seasonal allergy symptoms, stress incontinence in women, and cancer patients' nausea and vomiting. It may also help people with asthma feel better and ease their symptoms, but it hasn't been proven to make the lungs work better.[242]

Chiropractic[243]

A chiropractor uses their hands to help people who are having problems with their bones, muscles, or joints feel better.

---

[241] National Health System - https://www.nhs.uk/conditions/acupuncture (Reviewed in February 2023)
[242] NCCIH - https://www.nccih.nih.gov/health/acupuncture-what-you-need-to-know (Updated in October 2022)
[243] National Health System - https://www.nhs.uk/conditions/chiropractic (Reviewed in September 2023)

When muscles and joints hurt, chiropractors use a variety of methods, such as spine manipulation, short, sharp thrusting movements, moving your joints gradually into different positions, and pulling or stretching your muscles in different directions.
Most of the time, treatment doesn't hurt, but some people feel a little uncomfortable.
When done properly by a trained and licensed chiropractor, chiropractic care is usually safe.

The American College of Physicians run a systematic review of **low back pain** and found that exercise can help reduce this chronic pain, and spinal manipulation was better at relieving short-term pain than other active interventions.[244]
Unfortunately, there isn't much proof that it can help health issues that don't affect the muscles or joints.

Herbal medicines[245]

Medicines that come from plant parts, like leaves, roots, or flowers, are called herbal medicines, however, just because they are "natural" **doesn't mean they are safe**. Herbal medicines will have an effect on the body, just like regular medicines. If they are not used properly, they could be harmful. So, you should treat them with the same care and attention as regular medicines. Always let your doctor or pharmacist know about any plant medicines you're taking when you see them for health issues or are about to have surgery.
Unlike other medicines, not all herbal medicines are controlled, and there isn't a lot of proof that they work. Some people find them useful, but most of the time, their use is based on **old customs** rather than scientific study.

---

[244] Annals of Internal Medicine – https://www.acpjournals.org/doi/10.7326/M16-2367 (Published in February 2017)
[245] National Health System - https://www.nhs.uk/conditions/herbal-medicines (Reviewed in October 2022)

Blood and organs donation

Blood donation[246]

Safe blood **saves lives**. Women who are having problems during pregnancy or childbirth, children who are severely anemic (often from malaria or not getting enough food), accident victims, and people who have had surgery or cancer need blood. Transfusions save lives and make people healthier, but many people who need them can't get safe blood when they need it.

Blood can only be kept for a short time before it needs to be used, so there is always a need for a steady supply. Enough healthy people need to donate blood on a regular basis to make sure that blood is always available when and where it is needed.

The most valuable thing someone can give another person is blood. It gives life. Donating blood can save a life, or even more than one if the different parts of your blood (red cells, platelets, and plasma) are used separately to help people with different diseases.

Every year, about 118.54 million people give blood around the world, and a lot of these are taken in high-income countries, which are home to 16% of the world's people. From 2008 to 2018, there were recorded 10.7 million more blood donations from people who didn't get paid for them. 79 countries get more than 90% of their blood supply from unpaid, willing donors, while 54 countries, on the other hand, get more than 50% of their blood supply from paid or family/replacement donors.[247]

The blood service has to make sure that giving blood won't harm you, whether it's your first time or you do it all the time, as well as making sure that the person who receives your blood will be **safe** with it.

You will be asked about your medical history, including any medicines you are on and your present health before you give blood. You might

---

[246] https://www.who.int/news-room/questions-and-answers/item/blood-products-why-should-i-donate-blood (Published in June 2022)

[247] World Health Organization - https://www.who.int/news-room/fact-sheets/detail/blood-safety-and-availability (Published in June 2023)

also be asked about recent trips, for example if you live in a country without malaria, you might be asked if you have been to a tropical country lately.
Different people can give blood at different times, but most people can do so between the ages of 17 and 65.
Also, adults who are healthy can give blood often, at least twice a year.
Donating blood is not a good idea if you are sick, have anemia, are pregnant, have been pregnant in the last year, or are breastfeeding, have certain medical conditions that might make you an unsuitable donor, are taking certain medications like antibiotics, have or may have recently contracted an STD, have injected recreational drugs, have recently gotten a tattoo, skin scar or piercing.

It's very **easy** to give blood. Most of the time, giving blood takes 10 minutes, afterwards you can get back to your normal routine after sitting for 10 to 15 minutes and drinking some water. However, you should avoid doing anything too strenuous for the rest of the day. For the next 24 hours, you should drink a lot of water.
In most places, only 450 milliliters of blood are taken, which is less than 10% of your total blood volume.
Donating blood is very safe, and you almost never feel bad or have a problem during or after the donation.

Blood type is another thing to think about.
Blood types are based on whether certain antigens are present or not. These antigens are substances that can cause an immune reaction if they are not familiar to the body, so safe blood transfusions depend on careful blood typing and cross-matching because some antigens can make a patient's immune system fight the blood that was given to them.
Blood groups are based on whether 2 proteins, A and B, are present or absent on the surface of red blood cells. Besides the A and B antigens, there is a protein called the Rh factor that can be present (+ or positive) or missing (– or negative). This makes the 8 most common blood types: A+, A-, B+, B-, O+, O-, AB+, and AB-.

The most common blood types are O+ and A+, which respectively the percentage of donors are 37% and 30%; while the least common blood types are B-, AB+, and AB-, which percentages lower to between 1% and 2%.

Giving the right kind of blood can mean the difference between life and death.

People want types O- and O+ a lot. Even though only 7% of people are O-, there is a huge need for it because it is most often used during emergencies. People with blood type O- are called universal donors because their blood can be used to give to people of any blood type. From the other side, there is a high need for O+ because it is the most common blood type.[248]

Organ donation

There are 103,541 people on the national transplant **waiting list** in the US, and every day, 17 people die while waiting for an organ transplant. In 2022, more than 42,000 operations were done.[249]

Organ donations save or improve the lives of more than 3,000 people in the UK every year, but there are still about 7,000 people waiting for one. Every day, someone in the UK dies while waiting for a donation because not enough people are willing to give their organs.[250]

An organ donor can **save up to 9 lives** and make over 70 better.

You can choose not to be an organ and tissue donor when you die.

First, doctors and nurses will do everything they can to save your life, and only then they will think about organ giving.

---

[248] American Red Cross - https://www.redcrossblood.org/donate-blood/blood-types.html (Accessed in May 2024)

[249] Health Resources and Services Administration - https://www.organdonor.gov/learn/organ-donation-statistics (Reviewed in March 2023)

[250] NHS Blood and Transplant - https://nhsbtdbe.blob.core.windows.net/umbraco-assets-corp/30231/becoming-an-organ-and-tissue-donor-easy-read.pdf (Accessed in May 2024)

If you leave your organ donation choice on the record before you die, specialized nurses will check to see if you have made that choice.
Before you donate an organ or tissue, a specialist nurse will talk to your family or the person you chose, and they will be expected to back your choice. People are more likely to support organ giving if they know what their loved one wanted.
There aren't many ways for people to die so that they can be organ donors, consequently this means that the more people who sign up to be donors, the more likely it is that organ donation will be possible.

Some organs can be donated while the person is still alive, known as **living organ donation**, even if most organ and tissue gifts come from people who have already died.
You can give one kidney, one lung, a piece of liver, a piece of pancreas, or a piece of intestine while you are still living.

Stem cells donation[251]

Bone marrow is a remarkable factory. Blood stem cells live in the soft, squishy tissue in the middle of some of your bones, and these blood stem cells **make all of your important blood cells**, like white blood cells that fight infections and red blood cells that carry oxygen around your body.
Some illnesses, like some types of leukemia, make it impossible for the machine to work right, and for many of these people, getting a stem cell donation is their best chance of getting better.

One-third of patients have a sibling who is a good match, but the rest depend on the kindness of a stranger to give bone marrow or blood stem cells, and finding a good donor can be really hard. This is necessary because the donor and patient must have the same type of tissue (HLA - Human Leukocyte Antigen). Because there are so many possible combos of tissue types, we always need more donors, that's why it's so amazing

---

[251] NHS Blood and Transplant - https://nhsbtdbe.blob.core.windows.net/umbraco-assets-corp/19670/inf1326.pdf (Published in September 2020)

that you would be found as a possible match for a patient who needs you.
There are over 27 million donors on lists around the world, but this doesn't always work out. Each year, there is a 1-in-240 chance that a donor will come up as a possible match.
If a donor is found to be a possible match for a patient, the register will get in touch with him/her and ask for more blood samples so that they can do more tests to make sure it is a good match. Following these tests to see if he/she is a good match, there is a 1-in-5 chance that a donor will be asked to give to a patient.
In conclusion, as you may understand, it is **very unlikely** that donors will ever be called as a **possible match**.

As a donor, you may be asked to choose between **2 ways** to give stem cells.
Giving stem cells **from blood** that is already flowing is the first and most common way.
A nurse will come to your home or place of work 4 days before the donation and give you an injection of a drug that greatly increases the number of stem cells in your blood.
You will not need a general anesthetic on the fifth day while you will be hooked up to a cell-separator machine. Through a vein in one arm, the machine takes the stem cells out of your blood, and through a vein in the other arm, it puts the blood back into your body. If you have donated platelets before, you will know what this kind of machine does.
On occasion, you may be asked to come back on the sixth day to give more cells if the number you received is not enough.
The second way is to donate **bone marrow**, which means that stem cells are taken out of your hip bones.
This is done in a hospital with a needle and syringe while the person is asleep. Because the area where the needle was placed may get sore, you will need to stay in the hospital for up to 48 hours and then recover at home for up to 5 days.
You can donate stem cells in a hospital or center, and you can bring someone with you to help.

Even though stem cell giving is very safe, there are always some risks with medical procedures.
Both types of stem cell collection might make your bones hurt for a short time, but any small risks will be fully explained to you before you give.

Cord blood donation[252]

The blood that stays in the **placenta and umbilical cord** after giving birth is called cord blood, but most of the time, you throw away your placenta and the cord blood that is in it after giving birth.
There are a lot of **stem cells** in cord blood, and these cells can be used to treat many types of cancer, immune system problems, and genetic diseases.
The steps used to get cord blood are risk-free and safe for both the mother and the baby, because cord blood is taken from the placenta after the baby is born, the cord is cut, and the placenta is released.
Keep in mind that if delayed cutting was part of your birth plan, it may affect the chances of being able to collect the cord blood successfully. However, it is still possible to collect a useful amount of cord blood most of the time.
A lot of people can give their cord blood. To give cord blood, you must be at least 17 years old, and the medical staff has to make sure that every donation is as safe as it can be for the patient. To do this, they will ask the cord blood donors a series of questions about their health and lifestyle to make sure that every donation is safe for transfer.

[252] NHS Blood and Transplant - https://www.nhsbt.nhs.uk/cord-blood-bank (Accessed in May 2024)

Effects from Planet Earth pollution

Air contamination[253]

The world is getting hotter and more crowded, and our engines are still putting out dirty emissions. Since half of the world doesn't have access to clean fuels or technologies (like stoves and lamps), the air we breathe is becoming more and more polluted. In fact, 9 out of 10 people now breathe polluted air, which kills 7 million people every year.

Air pollution is **very bad for your health**; it's the cause of one-third of deaths from heart disease, lung cancer, and stroke. This is having about the same effect as smoking tobacco and a lot more than eating too much salt.

Sometimes it's hard to get away from dirty air, no matter where you live. It's everywhere. Air toxins that are very small can get through our bodies' defenses and hurt our lungs, heart, and brain.

Air pollution is closely linked to climate change - the main driver of climate change is fossil fuel combustion which is also a major contributor to air pollution - and efforts to mitigate one can improve the other.

The air is not healthy just because there is no smoke to be seen. The amount of harmful pollutants in the air in towns and villages around the world is higher than what the World Health Organization (WHO) says should be there every year.

---

[253] World Health Organization - https://www.who.int/news-room/spotlight/how-air-pollution-is-destroying-our-health (Accessed in May 2024)

The WHO, UN Environment, and the Climate and Clean Air Coalition's Breathe Life program made an online pollution meter to help people get a better idea of how dirty the air is where they live: check it out to https://breathelife2030.org/

Air pollution comes in 2 main forms: **ambient air pollution**, which is pollution outside, and **household pollution**, which is pollution indoor. The second one is about the smog that comes from burning fuels like coal, wood, or kerosene in homes that don't have enough air flow, like open fires or basic stoves. Because air goes from inside buildings to outside and back again, air pollution can be spread from inside to outside.
4 million people are killed every year by household air pollution. This is mostly a problem in Africa and Asia, where people use polluting fuels and technologies every day, especially for cooking, heating, and lights. Most of the damage is done to women and kids, who tend to stay at home more time.

The **main pollutants** are (1) particulate matter, which is a mix of solid and liquid droplets mostly released by burning fuel and cars; (2) nitrogen dioxide, which comes from cars or gas cookers inside; (3) sulfur dioxide, which comes from burning fossil fuels; and (4) ozone at ground level, which is made when sunlight reacts with pollutants from cars. Particulate matter, or PM, is the pollution that people are most affected by.

The most harmful particles are those with a diameter of 2.5 microns or less, because they can get deep into the lungs and stay there. These particles are very small, so they can get even into the bloodstream through the lungs, and they can make you more likely to get lung cancer, as well as heart and lung diseases.
Nitrogen dioxide and sulfur dioxide can also cause asthma, bronchial complaints, lung inflammation, and lessened lung function. Ozone is a major cause of asthma or makes it worse.

Children are severely hurt by air pollution. Up to 14% of kids between the ages of 5 and 18 around the world have asthma, which can be caused by things like air pollution. 543 000 kids younger than 5 years old die every year from lung diseases caused by dirty air. Cancers in kids are also linked to dirty air. Air pollution can affect the brain growth of a developing baby if it is breathed in by pregnant women. Children and adults both have trouble thinking and remembering things when they breathe in dirty air.

Air pollutants not only hurt our health, but they also damage the **environment** over time by causing climate change, which is itself a big threat to health and well-being.

There are mostly 3 **ways to avoid** taking in dirty air:

- Don't walk too far on busy streets during rush hour, and if you have a little one with you, try to keep it above vehicle exhaust.
- Don't spend too much time in places with a lot of traffic, like cars stopped at traffic lights.
- When you work out outside, try working out in places that are less dirty.

From the other side, these are the **ways you can fight** air pollution[254]

[254] World Health Organization - https://www.who.int/news-room/spotlight/how-air-pollution-is-destroying-our-health/10-ways-you-can-fight-air-pollution (Accessed in May 2024)

- Don't drive during rush hour; instead, walk to work, or take public transportation.
- Drive an electric car.
- Compost and recycle your trash. Don't burn it.
- Use renewable energy to run your home.
- Use less electricity.

In order to **reduce electricity usage** (and to pay less associated cost), first you need to know which are the top 5 energy consuming home appliances[255]

- **Wet appliances**: Washing machines, dishwashers, and dryers use the most energy (**14%** of the average bill). These home appliances use a lot of energy because they need to heat water, which makes them energy-hungry. You can use less energy by choosing to wash your clothes at a lower temperature, and to save water by not washing laundry in half loads. For your dishwasher, too, use the Eco setting if it has one and try to wait until it's full before starting it.
- **Cold appliances**: Fridges and freezers use about **13%** of the average home's energy. These machines have to be on all the time because that's how they work, so they're always using power to keep the temperature stable.
  Also, they're some of the most durable things in our house, taking an average of 17 years to break down, therefore it's a great idea to buy one that uses less energy because they'll be on all the time and could last all these years. When you buy a new fridge or freezer, think about both the smaller one that will work for you and the best-rated one that you can afford.
- **Consumer electronics**: That's not a surprise since consumer electronics like laptops, TVs, and game systems are so important to our daily lives these days. They make up about **6%** of your energy bill. Some of the oldest tips are still useful: remember to

[255] Energy Saving Trust - https://energysavingtrust.org.uk/top-five-energy-consuming-home-appliances (Updated in September 2023)

turn off standby mode on your devices when you're not using them.

- **Lighting**: The lights in your home use about **5%** of the total energy. If you replace your halogen lights with LEDs, you will use less energy.
- **Cooking**: About **4%** of your energy bill goes to running cooking appliances like the stove, oven, kettle, and microwave. Microwaves are more efficient than ovens because they only heat the food and not the air inside.

Ozone[256]

Between 15 km and 30 km above the earth, in the stratosphere, is the ozone layer, which **protects us** and all living things from the sun's dangerous ultraviolet radiation. Loss of the ozone layer could be very bad for both people and the world.

Because of ozone depletion, there is less shelter from the sun's rays and more exposure to **UVB radiation** at the Earth's surface. Over the course of a year, the ozone hole can cause the amount of UVB light to double at the surface in the Antarctic.

Studies in the lab and in the real world show that UVB causes non-melanoma skin cancer and is a major factor in the growth of malignant melanoma. Sunlight (UVB) has also been linked to cataracts, which are cloudy lenses in the eyes.

Stratospheric ozone is being depleted on both sides of the Earth, but this effect is stronger in the Southern Hemisphere (Antarctica) than in the Northern Hemisphere (Arctic). This process happens **more in the hemispheres** because the temperature of the atmosphere has a direct effect on how the ozone hole forms. When temperatures drop below -78°C, polar stratospheric clouds tend to form, which makes the loss of ozone worse. In the Antarctic, they form because of the long-term

---

[256] European Environment Agency - https://www.eea.europa.eu/en/topics/in-depth/climate-change-mitigation-reducing-emissions/current-state-of-the-ozone-layer (Modified in April 2023)

presence of low temperatures in the atmosphere, while in the Arctic, on the other hand, weather changes more from year to year.

As a result of the Montreal Protocol, which calls for the gradual removal of **Ozone-Depleting Substances (ODS)**, the ozone hole hit its largest size since 1979 in 2000.
Since 2001, when ODS emissions were stopped, the ozone layer has been slowly getting better, and the size of the ozone hole changes a lot from year to year because of the temperature in the stratosphere. For example, in 2019, warmer temps caused the ozone hole to be smaller.
As a whole, the efforts to stop ozone depletion are still very weak, and scientists say that more needs to be done to relieve the pressure that ODS put on the ozone layer.

Micro plastics[257]

In the past few years, a silent threat to health and the world has grown: microplastics, which are very small pieces of plastic less than 5 millimeters across. They are found in our seas, soil, and even the air we breathe. Because microplastics are **everywhere**, they are becoming a bigger problem for the environment and for people's health.
New research shows that people constantly breathe in and eat microplastics through contaminated seafood, like fish and shellfish. Microplastics have also been found in bottled water, tap water, and even drinks that most people drink, like beer and salt. A new study actually says that the average adult eats about 2,000 microplastics every year through salt.
A lot of different chemicals can get into our bodies through plastic water bottles, knives, and skin care products. There is evidence that these chemicals can cause major health problems, including problems with hormones, weight gain, insulin resistance, poor reproductive health, and even cancer.

---

[257] United Nations Development Program - https://www.undp.org/kosovo/blog/microplastics-human-health-how-much-do-they-harm-us (Published in June 2023)

What **effect** do microplastics have on human health, since smaller and smaller pieces of plastic are being found? What does this mean for our health? We still don't know.
Based on an analysis by the WHO, there isn't a lot of evidence to say that microplastics are having major negative effects on health right now. Scientists don't fully understand the effects of microplastics yet, and the data we have isn't strong enough to say for sure that they are harmful. More and better study is needed to get a more accurate picture of how people are exposed to microplastics and how they might affect health.

What **individuals and society can do** is to better handle plastics throughout the life cycle of a product and use less plastic when you can so that the plastics economy is more sustainable.

Antibiotics in livestock[258]

About 66% of all antibiotics used in the world are on farm animals, not on people. This is mostly used for everyday things, and it lets people keep farm animals (mostly pigs and chickens but sometimes also cattle) in bad conditions where diseases can easily spread. A lot of important groups, like the European Medicines Agency and the WHO, say that farming with too many medicines makes some human infections more resistant to antibiotics.

It is thought that **antibiotic resistance** will be a major problem for both people and animals in the future. More bacteria that are immune to antibiotics in the environment could make more infections that are not easy to treat. Some of the most common causes of death are bacterial diseases, and the way medicine is done today would be very different if there were no effective antibiotics.

[258] Alliance to save our antibiotics - https://www.saveourantibiotics.org/the-issue/antibiotic-overuse-in-livestock-farming (Accessed in May 2024)

Antibiotics have been used to raise animals for more than **50 years**, but in 2006, the EU banned their use for growth promotion. According to the World Organization for Animal Health, 108 countries no longer allow growth promotion, however, at least 40 countries still do.
A lot of drugs are still used in farming all over Europe, and farmers can even use antibiotics that the World Health Organization calls "highest-priority critically important" for people.
Antibiotics are also often given to groups of healthy animals in farms, even though they are used to treat sick people in conventional medicine, as more than 8 in 10 antibiotics used on farms in Europe are used for group treatments.
Europe has made some gains in the last few years, successfully dropping animal drug sales by a third from 2011 to 2018.

Pesticides[259]

Pesticides are used all over the world to keep bugs and other pests from damaging or destroying food. Pesticides that are no longer under protection, like dichlorodiphenyltrichloroethane (DDT) and lindane, can stay in the ground and water for years, but countries that signed the Stockholm Convention in 2001 have banned these chemicals. The Stockholm Convention is an international agreement that aims to stop or limit the production and use of persistent organic pollution.

How **dangerous** a chemical is depends on what it does and other things. To give you an example, insecticides usually hurt people more than herbicides. Different doses or amounts of a drug that a person is exposed to can make them feel different ways. Exposure way can also change how toxic it is, like if you swallow, breathe in, or come into close contact with the skin.
At the moment, **none** of the pesticides that can be used on food that is traded internationally are **genotoxic**, which means they damage DNA in a way that can lead to defects or cancer. There is a safe amount of

[259] World Health Organization - https://www.who.int/news-room/fact-sheets/detail/pesticide-residues-in-food (Published in September 2022)

exposure to these pesticides below which they don't cause harm. When people come into contact with **large amounts** of pesticide, they may become poisoned right away or have long-term health effects like cancer and problems reproducing.

People in low- and middle-income countries are more likely to die with pesticides than in high-income countries because people who come into close contact with pesticides are the most at risk, and these people include farmers who use pesticides and anyone else in the area during and right after the chemicals are spread.

Most people, who don't live in areas where pesticides are used, are exposed to much smaller amounts of pesticide residues in their food and water. On the other hand, people and the environment are still worried about the effects of chemicals.

One or more pesticides were found **above the levels** that would be considered dangerous at 22% of all tracking sites in rivers and lakes across Europe in 2020. A study done in 2019 found that 83% of farm soils tested had pesticide residues.

84% of people who took part in a large-scale human biomonitoring study in 5 European countries between 2014 and 2021 had at least 2 pesticides in their blood. Children always had higher amounts of pesticides than adults.

Pesticides are mostly ingested by most people because they stay on food, especially fruits and veggies but also meat and other animal products. They can also contaminate drinking water.

A new report from the European Food Safety Authority suggests that eating foods that contain certain pesticides probably won't hurt people's health. The method, on the other hand, did not consider the possibility of mixing effects. Maximum residue amounts were exceeded in only 1.7% of samples from Europe's most popular foods in 2020.[260]

[260] European Environment Agency - https
https://www.eea.europa.eu/publications/how-pesticides-impact-human-health
(Published in April 2023)

Technology

"It is not the strongest of the species that survives, nor the most intelligent, but the one most responsive to change"
Charles Darwin (Naturalist and geologist, circa 1800)

Apps[261]

As for the European Commission, **Mobile health** (also known as "**mHealth**") covers "medical and public health practice supported by mobile devices, such as mobile phones, patient monitoring devices, personal digital assistants (PDAs), and other wireless devices".
Personal guidance systems, health information and drug reminders sent via SMS, wireless telemedicine, lifestyle, and wellness apps that can

[261] Google Play and Apple Store (Accessed in October 2023)

connect to medical devices or sensors, like bracelets or watches, are all part of it.
As a new field that is growing quickly, mHealth has the ability to change the way healthcare is provided and make it better and more efficient.

In this chapter you can find the list of the most popular health apps for each category and function.
Since Apple Store does not disclose the number of downloads, you can find in this table only the downloads from Google Play platform, but this should still be an indicator of the app's popularity anyhow.

App	Downloads range (Millions)	Google Play / Apple Store rates	Developer
Leap Fitness Group – Fitness This company developed several fitness apps that got the highest downloads in this category. Here below there is the list of the most popular ones: • Home Workout - No Equipment • Six pack in 30 Days • Lose Weight App for Men • Workout for Women: Fit at Home • Height Increase Workout • Stretch Exercise - Flexibility	From 10 to 100	4.8 / 4.9	Leap Fitness Group
Step Counter – Pedometer This pedometer uses the built-in sensor to count your steps. No GPS tracking, so it can greatly save battery. It also tracks your burned calories, walking distance and	50	4.9 / 4.9	Leap Fitness Group

time, etc. All this information will be clearly displayed in graphs.			
Adidas Running Record your running sessions and review your statistics. Join challenges to get motivated – push your limits. Share your success with a global community and reach your goals with every step.	50	4.6 /	Adidas Runtastic
AllTrails Explore the outdoors: hiking trail maps, bike trails, camping & backpacking maps.	10	4.6 / 4.7	AllTrails
MyFitnessPal: Calorie Counter Track progress toward your nutrition, fitness, weight loss and water goals. This is an all-in-one food tracker, calorie counter, intermittent fasting tracker, macro tracker, and fitness tracker.	100	4.5 / 4.7	MyFitnessPal
Water drink reminder Water Drink Reminder reminds you to drink enough water. Proper hydration keeps your skin healthy and helps you lose weight.	10	4.8 /	Leap Fitness Group
Yuka Scan food and beauty products and evaluate their impact on your health	10	4.6 / 4.8	Yuka App
Flo Ovulation, period, and pregnancy tracker. Birth control pills and menstrual reminder.	100	4.6 / 4.8	Flo Health
Pregnancy + It features expert advice, daily	10	4.8 / 4.8	Philips Digital UK

articles, healthcare tips and interactive 3D models so you can track your baby's development.			
Baby + This app helps you to track your baby's growth, development, and upcoming milestones.	5	4.7 / 4.7	Philips Digital UK
Calm Tackle everyday stress and anxiety. Self-care and sound sleep through meditation.	50	4.2 / 4.5	Calm.com
Blue Light Filter - Night Mode Blue light filter is used to reduce blue light by adjusting the screen to natural color. Shifting your screen to night mode can relieve your eyes strain, and your eyes will feel at ease during night reading. Also, blue light filter will protect your eyes and help you sleep easily.	10	4.7 /	Leap Fitness Group
Blood Pressure App An assistant to help you to track your BP trends, find BP info and provide good lifestyle tips to benefit your health.	50	4.2 / NA	QR Code Scanner
Heart Rate Monitor - Pulse App Just put your fingertip on camera to get your heartbeat within a few seconds.	5	4.8 / 4.9	QR Code Scanner
NeuroNation - Brain Training Memory training and brain teasers to improve focus, logic, and memory.	10	4.6 / 4.6	NeuroNation
MyTherapy Pill Reminder A reminder for your medication, tablets, pills, and contraceptives	5	4.7 / 4.9	MyTherapy

Blood Sugar Tracker – Diabetes Smart blood sugar recorder is for you to log and analyze, preventing you from long-term health problems, and even improving your energy.	1	4.7 /	Leap Fitness Group
Manage My Pain The world's first and only commercially available digital chronic pain treatment companion with clinical validation and has one of the largest datasets for reported pain outcomes.	100k	4.7 / 4.2	ManagingLife
Ada – check your health One symptom checker for all your medical problems. Know and track your symptoms.	5	4.7 / 4.8	Ada Health
Habit Tracker - Habit Diary Feeling hard to break bad habits and build good ones? Habit tracker will bring you an easy and motivating habit-building journey.	5	4.8 / 4.7	Leap Fitness Group
First Aid American: Red Cross Stay safe during emergencies with expert tips & useful tools.	1	4.3 / 4.1	American Red Cross

Wearables[262,263]

The COVID pandemic sped up the use of wearable tech and made it more important in healthcare. People were already using wearables more because they liked the idea of keeping an eye on their own health

[262] Business Insider - https://www.businessinsider.com/5-examples-wearable-healthcare-devices-2021-5 (Published in May 2021)
[263] EduMed - https://www.edumed.org/spotlight/wearable-tech-smart-devices (Updated in January 2023)

before that, but in 2020, as new devices with better health-focused features hit the market, their use continued to rise.
We'll talk about some of the most popular wearable tech below.

Wearable fitness trackers: the sensors in these wristbands keep track of the users' heart rate and physical activity level. By connecting to different smartphone apps, many fitness trackers give you health and wellness advice. They might have a GPS built in, a heart rate monitor that works 24 hours a day, tracks stress and sleep, a relaxation breathing timer, and VO2 max data.

Smart health watches: smartwatches used to only be used to tell time and track steps, but now they can also be used as useful tools for healthcare. These smartwatches help people set goals for their workouts, track their mental health, remind them to move, check their blood oxygen level, and let them know if something is wrong.

Wearable ECG monitors: ECG monitors that you can wear are on the cutting edge of consumer tech. They can read electrocardiograms, or ECGs, which help people keep track of their heart rate and rhythm. They can also read other important signs, like blood pressure. Atrial fibrillation, bradycardia, tachycardia, heart pauses, and premature atrial contractions can all be found with these machines. Users can get results in 30 seconds by touching the bottom electrode to their left ankle or leg and placing their fingers on the top two electrodes. The monitor can also be worn as a chest strap, and it can be used with or without a smartphone.

Wearable blood pressure monitors: it checks blood pressure and tracks daily exercise, like how many steps you take and how many calories you burn. It finds the user's normal daily blood pressure and lets them know if their systolic blood pressure is 120 mmHg or higher.

Photoplethysmography (PPG) sensors: with PPG, doctors can find out how much blood is flowing to the heart in a non-invasive way. The

device uses a light sensor to track blood flow and help explain changes in heart rate. PPG sensors are smaller and easier to carry around than big ECG sensors that can be inconvenient. They also obtain information while the wearer is moving.
PPG devices are used to keep an eye on people who have high blood pressure, congestive heart failure, and other illnesses that cause blood flow problems.

Continuous Glucose Monitoring (CGM) sensors: tools that help people with type 1 diabetes keep an eye on their blood sugar levels 24 hours a day, 7 days a week. These monitors can also help people who need a lot of insulin, don't know if they have hypoglycemia, or have high or low blood sugar.
Most of the time, CGM devices are placed under your skin on your arm or stomach, and they have wireless receivers that send data to an outside monitor. Doctors and nurses use this data to change the medications they are giving.

Electronic skin patches: these patches stick right to the skin and are used to check vital signs, deliver medications, care for wounds, and sense motion. Electronic skin patches are a flexible form of wearable technology because they can be used for many things by healthcare workers.

Sweat and hydration sensors: athletes, people in the military, and workers can use sweat and hydration sensors to find out when they are exhausted, how much they are sweating, and how much water they need to stay healthy. Hydration and sweat sensors attach directly to the skin, and screens showing real-time updates that can be sent to a smartphone or similar device.
Hydration sensors can be used to keep an eye on people who are likely to become dehydrated or who have problems with their adrenal glands.

Wearable temperature monitoring: wearable temperature tracking devices give doctors useful medical information without the hassle of

measuring the temperature. They can be used to keep an eye on a baby's fever or do continuous, proactive COVID-19 diagnostics. Most of the products can be worn on the outside of the body without any problems, but some are meant to be implanted under the skin for more serious medical situations.
Core body temperature can tell also athletes a lot about how well they're doing.

Smart Wound Care: this wearable tech, which is also called "smart bandages," helps with wound care and healing by finding infections, releasing medications, and giving updates on progress. They are especially helpful for people who have long-term illnesses that leave wounds that won't heal.
Healthcare workers who treat people with diabetes, vascular diseases, obesity, and skin problems use smart wound care to help patients have better outcomes and cut down on the number of limbs that have to be amputated because of wounds that won't heal.

Monitors for pregnancy and birth: devices that pregnant women and babies can wear help find problems right away. Newborn monitors that are attached to a foot or ankle track breathing, sleep, and movement and send real-time reports. Pregnancy monitors send information about a fetus' heartbeat and movements continuously.
Doctors, neonatal nurses, and obstetricians use these tools to prevent needless stillbirth and injuries.

Smart contact lenses: smart contact lenses can help people who have lost or have trouble seeing in a number of ways. Augmented reality gadgets make pictures bigger and show them onto a smartphone so that they are easier to see. Other features check the amount of glucose in the blood, help people who are sensitive to light, and deliver medicine.
Optometrists use smart contact lenses to check on patients' eye health and find eye diseases earlier, as well as to improve their vision.

Smart glasses and head-mounted displays: virtual reality, augmented reality, eye trackers, and smart glasses could all help people who are losing their sight or having trouble seeing. These gadgets can change your life by helping you see again, making things bigger, increasing color contrast, or letting you use your voice to give instructions.

Wearable drug delivery: healthcare has put an emphasis on online care when it's possible as a way to deal with the COVID-19 pandemic. Wearable technology for drug delivery fits right into that story. Even though this technology isn't brand new, improvements in smart technology and delivery systems are making it possible to care for patients better, manufacture drugs, and find new ways to manage treatments.

Portable drug delivery technology has come a long way, and now there are subcutaneous devices, portable injectors, and needle-free injectors.

Smart clothes: by putting devices in underwear, clothes, and shoes, smart clothing could change the way healthcare is provided. These trackers record many kinds of biometric information, such as vital signs, heart rate, stress levels, and even information that can help with preventative health care.

As more smart clothing that can be worn becomes available, healthcare professionals will be able to collect useful data that will help them make earlier diagnoses and, eventually, stop deaths that happen because of late detection.

Wearable exoskeletons: the concept of medical exoskeletons that can be worn has been around for at least 100 years, but only in the last 30 years have there been huge steps forward that have turned this once-futuristic idea into a real medical possibility. A lot of people who have lost the use of their legs or are recovering from strokes or spine injuries use wearable exoskeletons to improve their quality of life. These goods can help people get their mobility back and are meant to improve both physical and mental health.

Wearable health alert and monitoring devices: the Centers for Disease Control say that every year, 1 in 4 people over 65 years old falls. Wearable health alerts and tracking devices make it easier for medical help to get to someone who needs it right away. The best devices are comfortable to wear, have long battery life, and are easy to use, and this is especially helpful for older people who want to stay independent while also making their loved ones' lives easier.

The most advanced devices can tell when someone falls or has a medical emergency on their own and send a warning to a pre-set list of caregivers, family members, and neighbors.

Biohacking[264]

According to the term "biohacking," there are many different tips and tricks that can help the body work better and maybe even make people live longer. Some types of biohacking may seem extreme, but others, like meditation and intermittent fasting, are pretty common and have been used for a long time, with a lot of study to back them up.

The act of using techniques from biology, genetics, neuroscience, and diet to improve health and well-being, boost mental or physical performance, or reach a specific health goal (like losing weight) is known as biohacking. Sometimes biohacking is also known as **Do-It-Yourself (DIY)** biology.

Virtually any method could be called biohacking if someone uses it to improve their biology in some way, so biohacking has a huge range of groups and options, almost too many to list.

Some people don't like biohacking because it's sometimes done "ahead of science," which means that people try hacks on themselves before they've been proven to work in a controlled clinical study setting. In fact, a 2020 article in the journal Science raised concerns about the lack of scientific oversight of many genetic biohacking and other DIY science projects that are now available to the public.

[264] Forbes - https://www.forbes.com/health/wellness/biohacking (Published in August 2023)

If you liked this book…

… please share your review on Amazon right now.

https://mybook.to/healthguide

This action will take you only a few seconds and it's fundamental for a book recognition, and therefore to potentially increase its popularity among the readers.
Let's say, in this way you can make your contribution in **spreading health around the world**!

Thanks in advance,

Lorenzo Valacca

Made in United States
Troutdale, OR
10/29/2024

24265401R00157